T0261940

Gangrene Management: Today and Tomorrow

Edited by **Tyler Smith**

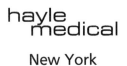

New York

Published by Hayle Medical,
30 West, 37th Street, Suite 612,
New York, NY 10018, USA
www.haylemedical.com

Gangrene Management: Today and Tomorrow
Edited by Tyler Smith

© 2015 Hayle Medical

International Standard Book Number: 978-1-63241-223-2 (Hardback)

Printed in the United States of America.

Contents

Preface

Gangrene is a major health concern and can cause adverse effects in its various clinical manifestations which result in considerable mass of body tissues dying due to some or the other cause. This book provides the readers with details on latest advancements and research in the field of gangrene management. It undertakes dialogues and discussions on clinical, physiological, bacteriological and other aspects of this method. Complicated challenges related to diabetic and non-diabetic gangrene management have also been extensively discussed. Specific interest has been taken to analyze current trends, as well as epidemiology of gangrene as a serious and potentially fatal complication.

This book unites the global concepts and researches in an organized manner for a comprehensive understanding of the subject. It is a ripe text for all researchers, students, scientists or anyone else who is interested in acquiring a better knowledge of this dynamic field.

I extend my sincere thanks to the contributors for such eloquent research chapters. Finally, I thank my family for being a source of support and help.

Editor

Impact Assessment of Diabetic Gangrene in Western Uganda

P.E. Ekanem, O.E. Dafiewhare, A.M. Ajayi,
R. Ekanem and E. Agwu

Additional information is available at the end of the chapter

1. Introduction

Diabetic gangrene is a chronic complication of diabetes which involves many medical, economic and social problems. It exerts a significant economic burden worldwide associated with high mortality (Hall et al., 2011) The surgical management of diabetic gangrene with limb salvage whenever possible accounts for huge expenditure in hospital practice, with long overall occupancy and considerable rehabilitation requirements (Vamos et al., 2010).

Historical background of this disease goes back to the 19th century and for much of the 20th century where it was conceptualized as 'gangrene in the diabetic foot' or as 'diabetic gangrene'(Connor, 2008). The prognostically and therapeutically important distinction between gangrene due to vascular insufficiency and gangrene due to infection in a limb with a normal or near normal blood supply was not made until about 1893(Connor, 2008).

Theoretically, diabetic gangrene is believed to most frequently affect digits of extremities. Gangrene of the lower limbs in diabetic patients and its malignant complication has been commonly reported (Gillitzer et al., 2004). Foot gangrene has also been reported to be 50 times more common in diabetic over the age of 40 than in non-diabetic of the same age (Gillitzer et al., 2004). Argawall et at. (2007) reported penile gangrene which may affect the prepuce and the glans penis. Fournier's gangrene is a rare, synergistic, fulminant form of necrotizing fasciitis involving the genital, perineal, and perianal regions (Eke, 2000). Fournier's gangrene is potentially fatal condition, affecting any age and gender, which results in thrombosis of small vessels, obliterated end arteries, and eventually skin and tissue necrosis (Yanar, 2006). Predisposing factors believed to contribute to the development of the disease are diabetes mellitus, alcoholism, malignancies, immunosuppression, liver, and renal disease (Kleemann et al., 2009).

The concept of the rising epidemic of diabetes mellitus and the observed increase of incidence of gangrene which has presented a substantial public health and socioeconomic burden in Sub-Saharan Africa has been widely reported (Mbanya et al., 2010). Diabetic neuropathy leads to a loss of sensation and subsequent alteration of the physical structure of the foot or any part of the body affected. The combination of tissue damage with increased susceptibility to infection in the foot leads to diabetic foot complications resulting in diabetic gangrene if not urgently managed. Interventions commonly employed in diabetic gangrene are limb salvage management and amputation which exert a lot of burden on the family and social institutions, that take care of this disability. Kidmas et al. (2004) in Nigeria reported 26.4% diabetic foot sepsis as one of the main indications for lower limb amputations. Agwu et al. (2010) reported 82% diabetic foot ulcers responsible for prolonged hospitalization of patients in South Southern Nigeria. Sié Essoh et al. (2009) reported 46.9% below knee diabetes related amputation and 11.2% below elbow diabetes-related amputations as common procedures performed in Ivory Coast (Cote D'Ivoire). However, in Zimbabwe, Sibanda et al. (2009) reported 9% diabetes related lower limb amputation rate among 100 patients evaluated

In the present context, Uganda has insufficient number of documented cases of diabetes care and even fewer data is available for diabetic gangrene among the diabetics. With increasing prevalence and interactions with other diseases, including the major communicable diseases in Uganda, diabetes is becoming a pressing public health problem.

1.1. Statement of the problem

Uganda is said to have 3.5% of its population as disabled (Monte, 2007) and extrapolated prevalence figure of 184,731 amputations annually (SCC, 2012). Unfortunately such data are lacking in highly systematic format that can give a picture of the contribution of diabetes gangrene to this number of amputations as in other developed countries. Economic cost of managing diabetes gangrene including limb salvage program, amputation and consequent disability is huge. If effective interventions are implemented in the near-future it may be possible to avert much of this burden, as primary prevention and treatment can reduce the incidence of both diabetic gangrene and a range of related diseases where diabetes is a causal factor. Information on the cost is lacking and yet critical for policymakers that can highlight the importance of introducing early and cost effective interventions for both primary and secondary preventions of diabetes gangrene.

1.2. The purpose of the study

The purpose of this study is to assess the impact of diabetes gangrene and its related complications among the diabetes in Western Uganda and the provision of relevant information for the planning of effective intervention for this disease.

2. Method

This was a retrospective evaluation of the impact of diabetes associated gangrene among patients in south western Uganda from May 2005 to July 2012. The seven years record of known diabetic patients clinically diagnosed with gangrene attending clinic in south western Uganda were assessed to determine the impact of diabetes, on the overall prognosis, disease induction, progression, management- including cost, prevention and control. Hospital records of diabetic patients attending clinics at Fort portal regional and referral hospital made available for this assessment were those confirmed by laboratory investigation and clinical observation which fulfilled our data inclusion criteria.

Thirty eight patients has been considered as qualified for inclusion in this study over the seven years study period. Fort Portal regional and referral hospital in south western Uganda was selected to act as sentinel collection center because it is known to see over 60% of hospital attendees in this region. Pre-tested semi-structured data extraction tools were used to extract data from the records of patients in the selected hospital. Focus group discussion and interview of participants in the study and available hospital health care providers were used to collect information not provided by the available case files and hospital record. Seventy three Health care providers that included clinical officers, nursing officers, laboratory technologists, staff found in the hospital record departments needed in the data extraction tool were used for this purpose.

Ethical approval was sought for and obtained from Kampala International University Ethical review committee. Informed consent of those who were interviewed was obtained and actual participants were assured of confidentiality of the information they provided.

3. Results

3.1. Result from data exraction tool

The demographic data extracted from the files of 38 patients studied showed 51.4% were males and 48.6% were females with ages ranging from 20-100 with a mean age of 59 as shown in table 1

Age(years)	Male (%)	Female (%)
20-40	4(11.4)	3(8.6)
41-60	5(14.3)	7(20)
61-80	7(20)	3(8.6)
81-100	2(5.7)	4(11.4)
Total	18(51.4)	17(48.6)

Table 1. Sex distribution of studied population

Several symptoms associated with gangrene as reported by the attending clinician include but not limited to: fever, loss of appetite and tachycardia (Table 2). Five percent (5%) of the patients who reported at the hospital diagnosed of dry gangrene manifested with fever and loss of appetite. The causes of dry gangrene in 5.3% of the patients were trauma and diabetes while

2.6% was caused by hematological disorders. Of those diagnosed with wet gangrene, 36.8% had fever and 7.9% was associated with loss of appetite while 5.3% had tachycardia as seen in table 2. Only 2.6% patients attending clinics for medical checkup were diagnosed of gas gangrene with tachycardia primarily caused by hematological disorders

Types of Gangrene	Associated symptoms			Primary cause of gangrene			
	fever	LA*	Tachycardia	trauma	diabetes	malignancy	HD*
Dry gangrene	2 (5.3)	2 (5.3)		2 (5.3)	2 (5.3)		1 (2.6)
Wet gangrene	14(36.8)	3 (7.9)	2 (5.3)	4 (10.5)	14 (36.8)	1 (2.6)	1 (2.6)
Gas gangrene			1 (2.6)				1 (2.6)

Table 2. Primary cause of gangrene and associated symptoms

LA* loss of appetite, HD* hematological disorders

From table 3 below, 2.6% of the patients diagnosed of dry gangrene came to the hospital with complications of retinopathy and neuropathy. It was later found that 2.6% of patients were alcoholics and smokers. 13.2% of those diagnosed of wet gangrene came to the hospital with complication of retinopathy, 5.3 % came with neuropathy, cardiomyopathy, nephropathy respectively, and 42.1% of patients diagnosed of wet gangrene were old, 5.3% had malnutrition problem, 2.6% were smokers and alcoholics respectively. There was no reported case of gas gangrene or its complications and no identifiable risk factors associated with it.

Type of Gangrene	Associated Complications of Diabetes					Risk Factors			
	Retino-pathy	Neuro-pathy	Cardio-myopathy	Nephro-pathy	Mal-nutrition	Old Age	smoking	Alcoholism	others
Dry Gangrene	1(2.6)	1 (2.6)					1 (2.6)	1 (2.6)	1 (2.6)
Wet Gangrene	5 (13.2)	2 (5.3)	2 (5.3)	2 (5.3)	2 (5.3)	16 (42.1)	1 (2.6)	1 (2.6)	13 (34.2)

Table 3. Associated complications of diabetes and risk factors in relation to different types of gangrene

In table 4 below, 71.1% of the patients clinically diagnosed with wet gangrene received antibiotics, 68.4% were given analgesics, 55.3% were given intravenous fluids, and 26.3% were given general treatment in line with the clinical judgment of the attending physicians because the patients complained of complex clinical signs and symptoms. None were on hyperbaric oxygen treatment. 50% of patients diagnosed with wet gangrene were amputated while in 18.4% debridement has been performed. 18.4% of those diagnosed with dry gangrene were given analgesics and antibiotics, 10.5% received intravenous fluid therapy, while none received hyperbaric oxygen treatment. In the group diagnosed with dry gangrene, 13.2% were amputated while in 2.6% debridement was performed.

2.6% patients diagnosed with gas gangrene all received analgesics, antibiotics, intravenous fluid, hyperbaric oxygen treatment respectively. None of them received any surgical treatment.

Type of Gangrene	Medical Management					Surgical Management	
	Analgesics	Antibiotics	I V fluids	Hyperbaric oxygen	Others*	Debridement	Amputation
Dry gangrene	7 (18.4)	7 (18.4)	4 (10.5)		1 (2.6)	1 (2.6)	5 (13.2)
Wet gangrene	26 (68.4)	27 (71.1)	21 (55.3)		10 (26.3)	7 (18.4)	19 (50)
Gas gangrene	1 (2.6)	1 (2.6)	1 (2.6)	1 (2.6)	1 (2.6)		

Table 4. Management pattern for the different types of gangrene

*Others: general treatment in line with the clinical judgment of the attending physicians

To have an insight into the magnitude of the surgical management of gangrene and associated cost, a survey of the level of amputation was noted as shown in table 5. It was observed, that 13.2% of those diagnosed with wet gangrene, received foot amputation, 10.5% were amputated below and above the knee respectively, while 5.3% were amputated below the elbow, including 2.6% who received above the elbow amputation as surgical treatment. No case of gas gangrene received amputation as a solution to their issues.

Table 5 also shows that 68.4% of participants with wet gangrene and 15.2% with dry gangrene attended the public section of Fort Portal Regional and Referral Hospital, because they wanted free treatment (probably explained by the fact that they belong to the low income class, living on less than one dollar a day as suggested by Agwu (2011). On the other hand, 10.5% patients with dry, wet and gas gangrene who attended private wing of the hospital, were able to pay from fifty thousand Uganda shillings to two hundred thousand Uganda shillings or twenty to eighty United states dollars [50,000 to 200, 000 Uganda shillings or US$20 to US$80 dollars] as cost for both medical and surgical management of the gangrene simply because they belong to the high income class living on above US$10 a day (Agwu, 2011)

Type of Gangrene	Level of Amputation						Cost (000 ug. /=)				Public
	Below Knee	Above Knee	Below Elbow	Above Elbow	Foot amputations	Others	<50	50-100	150-200	>200	
Dry Gangrene%		1 (2.6)	2 (5.3)		2 (5.3)					1(2.6)	6(15.2)
Wet gangrene %	7 (10.5)	4 (10.5)	2 (5.3)	1 (2.6)	5 (13.2)					2(5.3)	26(68.4)
Gas gangrene %								1(2.6)			

Table 5. Level of amputation and cost in different gangrenes

Type of Gangrene	Complications				Days on ward		
	Delirium	Circulatory ceasation	Post surgical sepsis	others	1-7 days	8-14 days	>14 days
Dry gangrene		1(2.6)			3(7.9)	1(2.6)	3(7.9)
Wet gangrene	2 (5.3)		1(2.6)		10(26.3)	7(18.4)	12(31.6)
Gas gangrene					1(2.6)		

Table 6. Post surgical complications and duration on ward for the different types of gangrene

Postsurgical complications noted from the files were delirium, circulation cessation on the limb, and post-surgical sepsis as shown in the table 6. Two patients(5.3%) having wet gangrene had delirium after surgery, one patient(2.6%) with dry gangrene had circulation cessation on the limb while another patient(2.6%) came down with sepsis. Table 6 shows that 5.3% of diagnosed with wet gangrene had delirium, and in 2.6% post- surgical sepsis had taken place.

Again 2.6% of those diagnosed with dry gangrene had circulation cessation on the limb. Wet gangrene generally caused certain delay in treatment and longer duration of hospital stay compared to dry gangrene and gas gangrene, as seen on the table. 31.6% of wet gangrene and 7.9% of dry gangrene were recorded as days spent above fourteen days.

	Type of amputation						Outcome			
	Below Knee	Above Knee	Below Elbow	Above Elbow	Foot amputation	Others	Escaped	Discharge	Death	Referral
Dry Gangrene (%)		1 (2.6)	2 (5.3)		2 (5.3)			6(15.8)	1(2.6)	1(2.6)
Wet Gangrene (%)	7 (10.5)	4 (10.5)	2 (5.3)	1 (2.6)	5 (13.2)		2(5.3)	12(31.6)	10(26.3)	
Gas Gangrene (%)									1(2.6)	

Table 7. Types of amputation and outcome for the different types of Gangrene

From table 7 above, Patients who were diagnosed with dry gangrene had (15.8%) discharge, one (2.6%) death and one (2.6%) referral. Of those patients who came to the hospital and were diagnosed with wet gangrene, twelve were discharged after surgery (31.6%), while ten (26.3%) died and two patients refused surgery. One of the patients diagnosed with gas gangrene died after surgery.

3.2. Result from interview

It was not clear why only 38 cases of diabetic gangrene were recorded over a period of seven years in retrospect from 2005 to 2012. To clarify this observation in relation to the current situation we organized a throughout participants' interviews and focused group discussion with available health care workers. Majority of the respondents alluded to the fact of poor storage and retrieval of files which led to missing files of the patients, resulting in the management asking patients to go with their files.

During the interview most of the stake holders agreed that based on their experience in the hospital, in the diabetic clinic, laboratory investigations and clinical examinations, that wet and dry gangrene with diabetes were the most often diagnosed gangrene in this region of the country. When asked whether gangrene treatment responds faster in patients with diabetes than non-diabetic, most answered no and asked to compare response to treatment with other diseases like HIV, cancer and sickle cell disease base on their experiences their responses were negative.

4. Discussion

There was a high incidence of diabetes-related gangrene in the western region of Uganda as seen in this study especially in wet and dry gangrene types. Comparatively, 36.8% gangrene cases due to diabetes, was far more than the 10.5% due to trauma, and 2.6% due to malignancy and hematological disorders. This shows that diabetic gangrene is the most prevalent condition, that sends people to the clinic for medical attention. Several reviews have described the frequent occurrence of gangrene, infection and sepsis associated with diabetic disease (Abbas, 2007) and with trauma to the hand (tropical diabetic hand syndrome) (Abbas, 2002) in Sub-Saharan Africa

The rate of undiagnosed diabetes is high in most countries of sub-Saharan Africa, and individuals who are unaware of the disorder, are at very high risk of chronic complications. Therefore, the rate of diabetes-related morbidity and mortality in this region could grow substantially. The observed high mortality in patients with diabetes and high prevalence of diabetes complications is likely to be a consequence of many late diagnosed and poorly controlled cases(Hall et al,. 2011). Assessing the public health importance of diabetes demands an appreciation of the impact of diabetes on other diseases and population mortality, and in particular the benefits of well-controlled diabetes for averting costly cardiovascular and microvascular complications (Kornum et al,. 2008 and Holman, 2008)

It is known, that several abnormalities of the host defense system might result in a higher risk of certain infections, including gangrene caused by diabetes. These abnormalities include immunological impairments, such as impaired migration, intracellular killing, phagocytosis, and chemotaxis of polymorphonuclear leukocytes from diabetic patients and neuropathic complications, such as impaired bladder emptying. In addition, a higher glucose concentration in the urine may create a culture medium for pathogenic microorganisms.

In most African communities, delivery of diabetes care is integrated into the overall national health-care structure. The idea of a specialized diabetes care centers and teams is plausible, however limited funding renders it impossible (Whiting et al., 2003). Health-care systems in most African countries are state-funded and priority is given to the unfinished agenda of communicable diseases. In most countries, including Uganda, there's limited free National Health Service; therefore, some patients may be treated free in the public unit of the facility while the private patients may enjoy some additional services. This was the case in Fort Portal regional and referral hospital where most of the diabetes related gangrene was treated in the public unit of the hospital free. In some cases the public unit may lack drugs and other facilities and when an individual with diabetes cannot afford the cost of drugs, the situation could be fatal (Beran and Yudkin, 2006). Several important challenges to accessing diagnosis and treatment have been identified in literature: the high financial cost of treatment, particularly that of insulin; the limited availability of diagnostic tools, treatment and glucose monitoring equipment; and a low awareness of diabetes among healthcare professionals (Beran et al., 2005). The total cost of these complications is likely to far outweigh the cost of effective primary and secondary prevention which is recommendable at this stage

In a region, where diabetes prevalence will double within the next 20 years, creation of a community-based system with appropriate financing should allow for cost-effective and rational use of limited resources. Meanwhile, in most rural and some urban African settings, health beliefs, knowledge, lay views, and health behaviour interact strongly (Kiawi et al., 2006, Awah et al., 2007). Due to misconceptions, indicated by popular health beliefs, many people in Africa fail to take proper measures for prevention and control of diabetes and its risk factors (Kiawi et al., 2006). Obesity is still seen as a sign of good living, because it confers respect and influence. Such lay perceptions are borne out of a contextual environment, in which most people are poor, hungry, and disadvantaged and, therefore, see obesity as a clear social marker for wealth (Renzaho, 2004). Persistent poverty and lack in much of sub-Saharan Africa means that traditional perceptions and cognitive imagery about lifestyle risk factors of diabetes are unlikely to alter in any important way, unless socio-culturally appropriate health promotion campaigns are implemented.

Gangrene has been a challenging public health issue for decades and continue to complicate already complex public health problems in developing and underdeveloped countries, including Uganda. The problem of case file storage and information retrieval as observed in this hospital opened our eyes to new area of challenge that could complicate effective management of gangrene in developing and underdeveloped countries. Other challenging factors include:

1.   limited resource to assist in prompt diagnosis and treatment,

2. poorly organized health systems, manned by low skilled healthcare providers,

3. poor up-take of health services by local dwellers, orchestrated by tradition, believes and demotivation due to low per capita income.

Poor information storage and retrieval can be explained by the facts that patients are still allowed to go home with their case files and to come back with them when next they need to see a health care provider. The authorities of the sentinel centers surveyed confirmed that such policy was practiced because there is poor attraction and retention of health workers at the rural communities thereby impacting on the capacity of the hospitals to maintain a system that would have accounted for all health issues in the hospital. This makes it difficult to control cases of dropouts where some patients who went home with their files never came back either because they are dead or moved to another location.

5. Conclusions

Diabetes gangrene has contributed to the high incidence of diabetes-related disability, morbidity and mortality in Uganda. The observed high mortality in patients with diabetes and high prevalence of diabetes complications is likely to be a consequence of many late diagnosed and poorly controlled cases. Hall et al. (2011) observed, that whilst epidemiological studies outside Sub-Saharan Africa have associated diabetes with infectious diseases of great importance in this region, the literature review identified little epidemiological data of this association in Sub-Saharan African countries like Uganda. This problem could have been contributed by poor information storage system identified in this study. Low skilled personnel who are demotivated due to low wages could not offer any new ideas on how to move the health system forward. Instead of being agents of change to optimize uptake of health services to the local communities, we found, that they themselves are victims of such factors as tradition, religious beliefs and demotivation among other factors which are known to dissuade people from utilizing the few available services in the communities. There is therefore a big gap between the available health care providers and locals who are supposed to reach out for the local communities.

Recommendations

Skill acquisition training workshops and health promotion to debunk erroneous ideas and beliefs surrounding diabetes gangrene are highly needed in Uganda. Anthropological perspectives are needed to elucidate the causes, prevention and control of diabetes, especially in Uganda as other African counties, where health outcomes are highly dependent on cultural variables. This in-depth qualitative research will inform stakeholders of the need for development and delivery of programs to prevent and treat diabetes and other chronic diseases, and will complement findings of quantitative epidemiological research. Multifaceted multidisciplinary research is also vital to clarify root causes and trends in the epidemiological transition of increasing diabetes in Africa

Author details

P.E. Ekanem[1], O.E. Dafiewhare[2], A.M. Ajayi[3], R. Ekanem[4] and E. Agwu[5]

1 Department of Anatomy, Kampala International University, Western Campus, Ishaka, Bushenyi, Uganda

2 Department of Internal Medicine, Kampala International University, Western Campus, Ishaka, Bushenyi, Uganda

3 Department of Pharmacology, Kampala International University, Western Campus, Ishaka, Bushenyi, Uganda

4 Department of Nursing Science, Kampala International University, Western Campus, Ishaka, Bushenyi, Uganda

5 Department of Microbiology, Kampala International University, Western Campus, Ishaka, Bushenyi, Uganda

References

[1] Abbas, Z. G, & Gill, G. V. Archibald L.K.: The epidemiology of diabetic limb sepsis: an African perspective. *Diabet Med* (2002).

[2] Abbas, Z. G. Archibald L.K.: Challenges for management of the diabetic foot in Africa: doing more with less. *Int Wound J* (2007).

[3] Agarwal, M. M, & Singh, S. K. Mandal AK: Penile gangrene in diabetes mellitus with renal failure: a poor prognostic sign of systemic vascular calciphylaxis. *Indian J urol* (2007).

[4] Agwu, E, Ihongbe, J. C, & Inyang, N. J. Prevalence of Quinolone susceptible Pseudomonas aeruginosa and Staphylococcus aureus in delayed-healing diabetic foot ulcers in Ekpoma Nigeria. Wounds (2010). , 4, 100-105.

[5] Awah, P. K, Kengne, A. P, Fezeu, L. L, & Mbanya, J. C. Perceived risk factors of cardiovascular diseases and diabetes in Cameroon.*Health Educ Res* (2007). PubMed, 25, 23-29.

[6] Beran, D, & Yudkin, J. S. Diabetes care in sub-Saharan Africa. *Lancet* (2006). , 368, 1689-1695.

[7]   Beran, D, & Yudkin, J. S. de Courten M: Access to care for patients with insulin-re-
      quiring diabetes in developing countries: case studies of Mozambique and Zambia.
      Diabetes Care (2005).

[8]   Chiang, I. N, Chang, S. J, Kuo, Y. C, Liu, S. P, & Yu, H. J. Hsieh J.T: Management of
      ischemic penile gangrene: prompt partial penectomy and other treatment options. J
      sex Med (2008).

[9]   Connor H: Some historical aspects of diabetic foot diseaseDiabetes Metab Res. Rev.
      (2008). Suppl 1:SS13., 7.

[10] Eke N: Fournier's gangrene: a review of 1726 casesBritish Journal of Surgery (2000).

[11] Ezera, A, & Ephraim, O. D. and Peter EE: Possible Diabetic-Foot Complications in
      Sub-Saharan Africa, Global Perspective on Diabetic Foot UlcerationsInTech, Availa-
      ble from http://www.intechopen.com/articles/show/title/possible-diabetic-foot-com-
      plications-in-sub-saharan-africa, (2011).

[12] Gillitzer, R, Franzaring, L, Hampel, C, Pahernik, S, Bittinger, F, & Thüroff, J. W. Com-
      plete gangrene of penis in a patient with arterial vascular disease. Urology. (2004). e
      4-6, 64, 1231.

[13] Holman, R. R. Year Follow-up of Intensive Glucose Control in Type 2 Diabetes. *N
      Engl J Med* (2008). , 10.

[14] Hall, V, Reimar, W T, & Ole, H. Nicolai L: Diabetes in Sub Saharan Africa 1999-2011:
      Epidemiology and public health implications. a systematic review. BMC Public
      Health (2011).

[15] Kiawi, E, Edwards, R, Shu, J, Unwin, N, Kamedjeu, R, & Mbanya, J. C. Knowledge,
      attitudes, and behavior relating to diabetes and its main risk factors among urban
      residents in Cameroon: a qualitative survey. *Ethn Dis* (2006). , 16, 503-509.

[16] Kidmas, A. T, Nwadiaro, C. H, & Igun, G. O. (2004). Lower limb amputation in Jos,
      Nigeria.*East Afr Med J.* , 81(8), 427-9.

[17] Kornum, J. B. Diabetes, glycemic control, and risk of hospitalization with pneumo-
      nia: a population-based case-control study. *Diabetes Care* (2008).

[18] Mbanya, J. C. N, Motala, A. A, Sobngwi, M. D, Assah, E, & Enoru, F. K. ST. ((2010).
      Diabetes in sub-Saharan Africa. The Lancet, , 375(9733), 2254-2266.

[19] Renzaho AMNFat, rich and beautiful: changing socio-cultural paradigms associated
      with obesity risk, nutritional status and refugee children from sub-Saharan Africa.
      Health Place (2004). , 10, 105-113.

[20] Shetty P: Diabetic Gangrene is CurableNational journal of homoeopathy (1998). vol.
      vii (3)

[21] Sibanda, M, Sibanda, E, & Jönsson, K. (2009). A prospective evaluation of lower ex-
      tremity ulcers in a Zimbabwean population. Int Wound J. 2009 Oct; , 6(5), 361-6.

[22] Sié EssohJ.B.; Kodo, M.; Djè Bi Djè, V. & Lambin, Y. ((2009). Limb amputations in
      adults in an Ivorian teaching hospital. *Niger J Clin Pract. 12* (3), 245-7.

[23] Vamos, E. P, Bottle, A, Edmonds, M. E, Valabhji, J, & Majeed, A. Millett C: changes in
      the incidence of lower extremity amputations in individuals with and without diabe-
      tes in England between 2004 and 2008. Diabetes Care. (2010).

[24] Whiting, D. R, Hayes, L, & Unwin, N. C. Diabetes in Africa: challenges to health care
      for diabetes in Africa. *J Cardiovasc Risk* (2003). CrossRef | PubMed, 10, 103-110.

[25] Yanar, H, & Taviloglu, K. Ertekin C: Fournier's gangrene: risk factors and strategies
      for management, World Journal of Surgery, (2006). , 30(9), 1750-1754.

Chapter 2

A Review of Clinical Manifestations of Gangrene in Western Uganda

Dafiewhare O.E., Agwu E., Ekanem P.,
Ezeonwumelu J.O.C., Okoruwa G. and Shaban A.

Additional information is available at the end of the chapter

1. Introduction

1.1. Definition

Gangrene is described as the necrosis or death of soft tissue due to obstructed circulation, usually followed by decomposition and putrefaction (Vitin 2011).

It may also be defined as irreversible tissue or organ death caused by loss of blood supply to the affected area. It is a serious and potentially life-threatening medical condition that has significant economic burden worldwide [Hall et al., (2011)].

1.2. Etiology and risk factors

Gangrene is primarily caused by diminished or total loss of blood supply to body tissues that leads to cell death. The compromised blood supply may result from trauma, serious injury, surgery, infection or chronic vascular diseases and immunosuppression. Other risk factors include diabetes mellitus, human immunodeficiency virus infection, long term smoking, alcoholism, malignancies, liver and renal diseases [Czymek et al., 2009]. Multiple digital gangrene has been reported to result from traditional therapy [Unuigbe et al., 2009].

1.3. Prevalence and incidence

The prevalence and incidence of gangrene are difficult to establish [Vivek, 2011] because some patients may die from gangrene and its complications without visiting healthcare facilities, especially among poor rural dwellers with few or no healthcare facilities. For example, though Fournier's gangrene has been widely reported to be commoner among males [Ndubisi and Raphael 2011, Kim 2011 and David 2011], Czymek et al (2009) found Fournier's gangrene to be more common in females. Among those who visit health centres, the diagnosis may be missed and when diagnosed correctly, it may not be recorded in patients' hospital records. A patient's operation notes may capture gangrene, but the main operating theatre registration book and ward records may only reflect titles like intestinal obstruction, exploratory laparotomy, acute abdomen, etc. In addition, the prevalence and incidence of gangrene are closely related to the known causes and risk factors. These are chiefly non-communicable diseases (NCDs) like chronic cardiovascular diseases (e.g. arteriosclerosis) and diabetes mellitus. There is high prevalence of people with NCDs [Agwu et al (2011)] who do not know that they have the diseases. Such people have higher risk of developing complications associated with the NCDs and one of such complications is gangrene. Gangrene can affect all age groups and sexes.

1.4. Types

There are two major types of gangrene – dry and wet gangrene [Charles 2012]. Gas gangrene, sometimes listed as a third type of gangrene in some texts is actually a type of wet gangrene. Other types of wet gangrene include necrotizing fasciitis and internal gangrene. Gangrene may affect superficial (in the skin or near the skin) or deep tissues (beneath the skin). Superficial gangrene often affects distal parts of the body like toes and fingers. It can also affect the penile shaft or scrotal skin. However, gangrene can also affect deep body tissues and organs.

1.5. Clinical manifestations

Gangrene may be diagnosed from its clinical manifestations, especially when it affects superficial body parts. However, gangrene affecting deep tissues may sometimes be difficult to diagnose from clinical manifestations. Some cases of gangrene are diagnosed at surgery e.g. gangrenous bowel loop. The clinical manifestations of gangrene depend on a number of factors which include type of gangrene, location in the body, cause and underlying disease processes in the affected person [Charles 2012]. Early diagnosis of gangrene is important in curbing local disease progression and its systemic complications which are often fatal. Though superficial gangrene may be easily diagnosed by clinicians, some people are unaware they live with it. Some present with other medical conditions and their gangrene is diagnosed incidentally.

1.6. Treatment

The definitive treatment for gangrene is surgical excision of the affected tissues. Where distal extremities like toes, fingers or distal parts of the lower limbs are affected, the treatment is amputation. However, when deep tissues like intestines are gangrenous, bowel resection and anastomosis is done. Though this may not leave the patient with a physical disability, functional challenges sometimes develop, especially when long lengths of bowel are resected. Awori and Atinga in 2007 reported that diabetes-related gangrene alone accounted for 17.5% of patients who underwent amputation in Kenya. Penectomy has been reported for penile gangrene [Chiang *et al.* 2008].

2. Problem statement

The prognosis of gangrene is highly dependent on early detection of its clinical manifestations, diagnosis and institution of appropriate treatment. Early detection of clinical manifestations of gangrene remains a challenge to healthcare providers due to limited resources. There was therefore a need to document the practical clinical manifestations of gangrene in South-Western Uganda so that evidence based data-base could be generated for use in gangrene diagnosis with the ultimate goal of improving the current capacity to diagnose gangrene in resource limited settings. In this chapter, we therefore focused on how gangrene manifests in South-Western Ugandan communities.

3. Objectives and relevance

In this chapter, we documented the clinical presentations of gangrene in medical records of patients who were diagnosed and managed for gangrene in South Western Uganda from May 2010 to April 2012. Ultimately, this chapter was aimed at alerting health-workers on how gangrene manifests in our practice area and helping promotion of its early diagnosis. This information shall hopefully open new grounds for further research on how patients with gangrene present to healthcare institutions and promote health education that can lead to reduction in the prevalence of gangrene.

4. Methodology

4.1. Study area

Bushenyi, Sheema and Rubirizi Districts of South Western Uganda were chosen for this study. The biggest hospital in each of the three Districs were chosen because they receive the highest number of patients in each of the Districts. These hospitals were Kampala International University Teaching Hospital (KIUTH), Kitagata Hospital (KH) and Rugazi Health Centre (RHC). These sites were carefully selected to represent the varied diversities present in the region. Also, they were selected because they provide free medical healthcare services and they are patronized by many members of the community. They also receive referrals from lower government owned and private healthcare units. In addition, KIUTH is one of the major referral centers in the region that receives patients directly from her community and referrals from many healthcare units within and outside the western region, including neighboring countries like Democratic Republic of Congo and Rwanda.

4.2. Ethical considerations

Ethical clearance was obtained from the Institutional Research and Ethics Committee of Kampala International University before the study was commenced. Permission to access the files of patients was sought and obtained from the heads of each health facility used. The heads of the hospitals were assured of confidentiality of their patients' identity and only the data without their identity would be published for knowledge transfer and research purposes.

4.3. Sample Size

Medical records of all patients diagnosed to have gangrene within the selected health facilities from May 2010 to April 2012 were used for the study.

4.4. Inclusion criteria

All patients' medical records that had the term "gangrene" in the diagnosis(es) and differential diagnosis(es) within the study timeframe were included.

4.5. Exclusion criteria

All medical records that did not have the term "gangrene" in their diagnosis(es) and differential diagnosis(es) were excluded.

4.6. Data collection instruments

Data sheets were designed and used for the study. They were pre-tested at KIUTH for validity before using them for the study. The research instruments were designed for collection of both qualitative and quantitative data. The data collected included variables like age, sex, education level, occupation, complaints, duration of complaints and treatment received before visiting healthcare facility. Others included type of gangrene and disclosure of diagnosis to patients by hospital staff.

5. Data collection

5.1. Data collection procedure

Hospital file numbers of all patients whose diagnosis(es) contained the word "gangrene" from May 2010 to April 2012 were retrieved from all ward registers of each participating hospital. The case notes/folders were retrieved from the medical records departments of each hospital. Data from patients' records were retrieved by researchers using data sheets.

5.2. Data quality control

All data collection procedures were done by members of the research team. At the end of each data collection session, all members of the research team met to review and resolve challenges encountered during the data collection process. The final data were manually entered into Microsoft Excel 2010 package for data analysis.

6. Results

We found a total of 22 patients' case notes/folders that met our inclusion criteria. There were 15, 4 and 3 from KIUTH, KH and RHC respectively. There were 9 cases of dry gangrene and 13 were wet gangrene. Among the wet gangrene cases, 10 started as wounds that later became infected, while 3 started spontaneously and were diagnosed to be Fournier's gangrene. Details of the results are displayed in the tables below.

INSTITUTION	FREQUENCY	PERCENTAGE (%)
KIUTH	15	68.2
KH	4	18.2
RHC	3	13.6
TOTAL	22	100.0

Table 1. Number of patients with gangrene per healthcare unit

The highest percentage (68.2%) of cases was found in KIUTH followed by KH (18.2%) and then RHC (13.6%) as shown in table 1.

SEX	FREQUENCY	PERCENTAGE (%)
MALE	14	63.6
FEMALE	8	36.4
TOTAL	22	100.0

Table 2. Sex distribution of patients

Table 2 above shows that more males (63.6%) suffered from gangrene, compared to 36.4% seen among females.

TYPE OF GANGRENE	FREQUENCY	PERCENTAGE (%)
DRY	9	40.9
WET	13	59.1
TOTAL	22	100.0

Table 3. Type of gangrene

Table 3 above shows that there were more cases of wet gangrene in the communities studied.

RESPONDENTS' AGE IN YRS	FREQUENCY	PERCENTAGE (%)
<20	3	13.6
20 - 29	3	13.6
30 - 39	6	27.3
40 - 49	3	13.6
50 - 59	5	22.7
60 - 69	0	0.0
70 - 79	1	4.6
80 - 89	0	0.0
>90	1	4.6
TOTAL	22	100.0

Table 4. Age distribution of patients with gangrene

Table 4 above shows that most patients (27.3%) with gangrene were aged between 30 and 39 years. The next age was those between 50 and 59 years (22.7%).

The age distribution of patients affected by gangrene is presented in Figure 1 below. It gives a pictorial view of the age distribution of patients that bear the burden of gangrene.

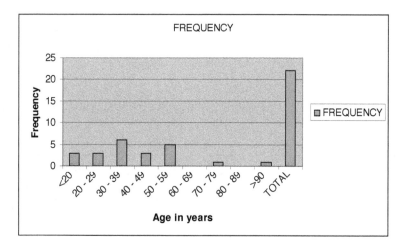

Figure 1. Histogram of Age distribution of patients with gangrene

OCCUPATION	FREQUENCY	PERCENTAGE (%)
STUDENT	3	13.6
TEACHER	1	4.6
FARMER	11	50.0
BUSINESS PERSON	3	13.6
UNKNOWN	4	18.2
TOTAL	22	100.0

Table 5. Occupation of patients with gangrene

Table 5 above shows that most of the patients (50%) that suffered from gangrene were farmers.

COMPLAINT	FREQUENCY	PERCENTAGE (%)
PAIN	20	42.6
LOCAL SWELLING	18	31.9
WOUND	6	12.8
UNCONSCIOUSNESS	3	6.4
UNKNOWN	3	6.4
	47	100.0

Table 6. Presenting complaints of patients with gangrene

Table 6 above shows the main complaints that patients with gangrene reported at the time of visiting the healthcare units. Pain was the commonest complaint (42.6%), followed by local swelling (31.6%) and wounds (12.8%). The 3 patients (6.4%) that were brought to hospital in coma were all diagnosed to have diabetes mellitus.

PREVIOUS TREATMENT	FREQUENCY	PERCENTAGE (%)
YES	8	36.4
NO	14	63.6
TOTAL	22	100.0

Table 7. Previous treatment received by patients with gangrene before visiting healthcare unit

DIAGNOSIS DISCLOSED TO PATIENTS	FREQUENCY	PERCENTAGE (%)
YES	21	95.5
NO	1	4.6
TOTAL	22	100.0

Table 8. Diagnosis disclosure by healthcare staff to patients

Disclosure of information regarding the diagnosis by healthcare workers to the patients was noted to be very encouraging. 95.5% of the patients admitted that they were informed about the diagnosis made by the clinicians.

DURATION OF SYMPTOMS IN MONTHS	FREQUENCY	PERCENTAGE (%)
≤ 1	12	54.6
≤ 2 and > 1	3	13.6
≤ 3 and > 2	1	4.6
≤ 4 and > 3	0	0.0
≤ 5 and > 4	1	5.6
≥ 5	5	33.7
TOTAL	22	100.0

Table 9. Duration of symptoms before presentation to healthcare unit

This study revealed that most patients (54.6%) with gangrene lived with symptoms for one month or less. The figures are shown clearly in Table 9 above.

MANIFESTATION CHANGES	FREQUENCY	PERCENTAGE (%)
YES	5	22.7
NO	17	77.3
TOTAL	22	100.0

Table 10. Changes in clinical manifestations before visiting healthcare unit

Table 10 above shows that majority (77.3%) of those studied did not notice major changes in the clinical manifestations of gangrene from the time of onset till the time they visited hospital for care.

7. Discussion

Gangrene is one of the Non-Communicable Diseases (NCDs) contributing to the morbidity and mortality burden of people in Uganda and Africa in general. The diagnosis of gangrene is made by clinicians in our community, but there is a lot of under-recording in health records. This occurs more commonly among patients with gangrene affecting internal tissues/organs. This has made gangrene not to occupy a prominent position in health reports from Uganda and other parts of the world. It is believed that the situation is similar in many other African countries and beyond. The reality of gangrene only becomes manifest when patients with superficial or peripheral gangrene manifestations are faced with the option of giving informed consent for amputation. This is usually a very challenging moment for patients and their close relatives. In some cases, there is delay in instituting the definitive care (i.e. amputation) due to time required to give adequate counseling to patients and their relatives before they can accept surgery. The economic burden associated with management of gangrene and the post-operative social consequences that result affect patients and relatives' negatively in diverse ways. One such complication is stump wound infection. Obalum and Okeke 2009 reported 26.5% stump wound infection in Nigeria. Surgical care for gangrene accounts for huge financial cost in hospital practice, long hospital stay and significant rehabilitation requirements [Vamos *et al.*, 2010].

It is common knowledge that gangrene is caused by loss of blood supply to tissues. Many causes of blood supply loss are known and preventable. Therefore gangrene can be prevented in many instances. However, when prevention fails, gangrene's debilitating effects can be reduced in many cases if the symptoms and signs are detected early. Early detection and institution of treatment is one of the major ways of reducing morbidity and mortality associated with diseases generally and this is applicable to gangrene. Despite the available knowledge to us today, many people in our community still suffer by living with gangrene for prolonged periods before presenting to healthcare centres for attention.

The results showed that all the patients seen were either incidentally diagnosed to have gangrene or came to the healthcare units to seek medical attention because of worsening condition of their wounds. The results revealed that the highest percentage of cases was found in KIUTH followed by KH and then RHC (Table 1). This was not a surprise, because KIUTH is the biggest and only teaching hospital in the three Districts studied. It also receives referrals from more health units than the other two put together.

From table 2, it was observed that more males (63.6%) had gangrene compared to females. This might have been due to the fact that males do more activities that predispose them to sustaining injuries like farming and technical works.

Table 3 shows a higher prevalence of wet gangrene in the communities studied than the dry gangrene. In essence, this might be a true reflection of the prevalence.

In table 4, it can be seen that the age group that was most affected by gangrene was 30-39 years, followed by 50-59 years and then 20 -29 years; entailing that these are the most active and productive age groups in any community and therefore will often exert a far-reaching economic and administrative impacts on their respective communities.

Table 5 reveals a higher prevalence of farmers being affected by gangrene. The Districts are mainly occupied by peasant farmers. However, it must be noted here that some of the patients may not have been farmers, because in practice, we find that some traders introduce themselves as farmers in this region since farming is the major occupation of the people.

Table 5 reveals a higher prevalence of farmers being affected by gangrene. The Districts are mainly occupied by peasant farmers. However, it must be noted here that some of the patients may not have been farmers, because in practice, we find that some traders introduce themselves as farmers in this region since farming is the major occupation of the people.

Table 6 shows the main complaints that patients with gangrene reported at the time of visiting the healthcare units. Pain was reported to be the commonest complaint of patients followed by local swelling and then wounds. Three patients (6.4%) were brought to hospital in coma and were all diagnosed to have diabetes mellitus.

From table 7, it was observed that the majority of the patients did not visit any other places to seek medical attention before presenting at the highest hospital in their respective Districts. This might be due to information that they got from staff members of the major hospitals on their usual visits for health talks and home visits in some of the hard-to-reach villages where some of the patients live. It could also have been that those who presented for the first time in the hospitals studied might have had serious pain that they believed could only be managed at the best health facilities nearest to them in the shortest time possible.

In table 8, disclosure of information regarding the diagnosis by healthcare workers to the patients was almost a hundred per cent. This good practice should be encouraged because when patients are well informed about their diagnosis(es), they are empowered to contribute more meaningfully towards the choice of treatment that they eventually receive.

It is noted from this study that most patients with gangrene lived with symptoms for less or equal to one month. The figures are shown clearly in Table 9 above. This might have been due to the discomfort associated with the symptoms they had. It is believed that the three main symptoms that made them to present within the short timeframe were pain, swelling and foul-smelling wounds from Table 6 earlier discussed above.

Table 10 above shows that majority of those studied did not notice major changes in the clinical manifestations of gangrene from the time of onset till the time they visited hospital for care. This is most likely due to the fact that majority of them presented within the first month of onset of the disease. The 5 (22.7%) patients who noted changes in the clinical manifestations before visiting hospitals most likely had dry gangrene which they were able to live with for longer periods. We note that in Table 10 (Changes in clinical manifestations) did not tally with the figure in Table 3 (Type of Gangrene). We believe that several factors might have been responsible for the variation and such factors might include presence of multiple pathology or co-existence of wet and dry gangrene in the same patient in the same location at the same time.

Generally, most of these patients had believed that their leg ulcerations were just like common wounds that heal with time. Even those who noticed darkening of the skin over their toes following tissue death did not know that the affected toes were no longer functional until they were informed by their clinicians. They were able to cope with pain in most cases, hence some of them presented late to hospital. However, some patients had severe excruciating pain that prompted them to even plead with the surgeons to amputate the affected limb in extreme cases.

The health burden associated with gangrene can be minimized if its clinical features are well known to both healthcare workers and the public. As noted earlier, manifestations of the gangrene depend on several factors, including the type, cause, location in the body and associated underlying diseases.

Often, dry gangrene begins with the affected area first becoming numb and cool. The pain experienced depends on patients' pain threshold. The affected area then changes colour, usually turning from reddish to brownish and eventually blackish. While the above processes are taking place, the local area also shrinks and becomes dry. Dry gangrene resulting from immediate arterial blood loss may first turn pale or bluish before progressing as described above [Charles 2012].

On the other hand, wet gangrene commonly starts with swelling and severe pain in the affected area which may be initially red. Putrefaction evidenced by sloughing tissue, pus, local oozing of fluid may follow, associated with a foul odour produced by the infectious agent(s) that destroy(s) the tissues. Both dead and dying tissues later become moist and develop black appearance that is pathognomic of gangrene. Other systemic symptoms often seen in patients with wet gangrene include fever and other signs of severe systemic disease.

It must be noted here that clinicians need to have a high index of suspicion when examining patients that have a high risk of developing gangrene e.g. diabetics, chronic cigarette smokers and immune-compromised patients. Others include patients with chronic ulcers and those with known chronic cardiovascular diseases associated with poor vascular perfusion. It must be noted here that though many people present with the usual classical triad of polyuria, polydipsia and polyphagia, some patients with diabetes mellitus present with coma as the first symptom. This suggests that many more people are quietly living with diabetes mellitus in the communities. If such people are not diagnosed through pragmatic efforts by Government, Non-Governmental Organizations and well-meaning members of the society, the increase in gangrene resulting from diabetes mellitus alone shall continue to rise rapidly in Western Uganda.

All the reports documented in this study have been on superficial or peripheral gangrene. Deep soft tissue gangrene were missed because of the exclusion criteria used that stated that only patients whose diagnosis(es) and/or differential diagnosis(es) clearly included the word "gangrene" were to be used. The figures reported are therefore far below what truly exists in our community. Thus, there is need to critically address the problem of under-reporting in healthcare/health ministry and other ministries in Uganda and other African countries. Special attention needs to be given to surgical findings from our operating theaters in the final documentation of diseases in all patients' hospital records to enable health planners make proper plans for the people they serve.

8. Conclusions/recommendations

This study has shown that the prevalence of gangrene remains unknown in our community. The report is definitely a tip of the ice-berg regarding the disease burden of gangrene in Western Uganda. Though the numbers are few, the burden is much for anyone that suffers from gangrene. Since the clinical manifestations of deep tissue gangrene may be vague, clinicians are encouraged to have a high index of suspicion in all patients that have risk factors for developing gangrene at any clinician-patient consultation to promote early detection and institution of appropriate preventive and curative measures.

It is also recommended that findings seen during surgical operations should be documented adequately, included in patients' diagnoses and health records as these will reduce the much talked about under-reporting syndrome in developing countries, including Uganda.

Finally, it is recommended that further local prospective studies should be done for longer periods and in more places in Uganda in order to be able to document the true prevalence of gangrene and their clinical manifestations among members of our community. It is believed that such studies shall reveal how early signs and symptoms manifest among Ugandans and other parts of the world.

9. Study limitations

The major limitation of the study was poor documentation of medical findings and poor record keeping. Poor documentation manifested as absence of the term "gangrene" in many patients' records e.g. bowel loop gangrene where diagnoses were simply recorded as acute abdomen or exploratory laparotomy etc.

Acknowledgements

We wish to acknowledge the management and staff members of Kampala International University Teaching Hospital, Kitagata Hospital and Rugazi Health Centre that supported us by releasing relevant data used for this study. In particular, we acknowledge the support given to us by our family members during the time we had to travel out of station to gather information and the late nights we spent away from them while preparing this document.

Author details

Dafiewhare O.E.[1], Agwu E.[2], Ekanem P.[3], Ezeonwumelu J.O.C.[4], Okoruwa G.[5] and Shaban A.[6]

1 Department of Internal Medicine, Kampala International University, Western Campus, Ishaka, Bushenyi, Uganda

2 Department of Microbiology, Kampala International University, Western Campus, Ishaka, Bushenyi, Uganda

3 Department of Anatomy, Kampala International University, Western Campus, Ishaka, Bushenyi, Uganda

4 Department of Clinical and Bio-pharmacy, Kampala International University, Western Campus, Ishaka, Bushenyi, Uganda

5 School of Pharmacy, Kampala International University, Western Campus, Ishaka, Bushenyi, Uganda

6 Department of Surgery, Kampala International University, Western Campus, Ishaka, Bushenyi, Uganda

References

[1] Vitin A.A., editor. Gangrene - Current Concepts and Management Options. Rijeka: InTech; 2011. http:// www.zums.ac.ir/files/research/site/medical/Surgery/ Gangrene_Current_Concepts_and_Management_Options.pdf (accessed 20 December 2012).

[2] Awori, K.O and Atinga, J.E.O. (2007). Lower limb amputation at Kenyatta National Hospital Nairbi. *East Afr J*. 84:121-126.

[3] Charles P.D. Gangrene at a glance. http://www.medicinenet.com/gangrene/article.htm (accessed 28 September 2012).

[4] Chiang I.N, Chang S.J, Kuo Y.C, Liu S.P, Yu H.J, Hsieh J.T. Management of ischemic penile gangrene: prompt partial penectomy and other treatment options. J sex Med 2008, 5(11):2725-33.

[5] Czymek R, Hildebrand P, Kleemann M, Roblick U, Hoffmann M, Jungbluth T, Bürk C, Bruch HP, Kujath P. New insights into the epidemiology and etiology of Fournier's gangrene: a review of 33 patients. Infection. 2009 Aug;37(4):306-12. Epub 2009

Jul 23. Available at http://www.ncbi.nlm.nih.gov/pubmed/19629386. (accessed 29 September 2012).

[6]   David Kearney (2011). Fournier's Gangrene: Diagnostic and Therapeutic Considera-
      tions, Gangrene - Current Concepts and Management Options, Alexander Vitin
      (Ed.), ISBN: 978-953-307-386-6, InTech, Available from: http://www.intechopen.com/
      books/gangrene-current-concepts-and-management-options/fournier-s-gangrene-di-
      agnostic-and-therapeutic-considerations (accessed 28 September 2012).

[7]   Ezera Agwu, Ephraim O. Dafiewhare and Peter E. Ekanem (2011). Possible Diabetic-
      Foot Complications in Sub-Saharan Africa, Global Perspective on Diabetic Foot Ul-
      cerations, Dr. Thanh Dinh (Ed.), ISBN: 978-953-307-727-7, InTech, Available from:
      http://www.intechopen.com/books/global-perspective-on-diabetic-foot-ulcerations/
      possible-diabetic-foot-complications-in-sub-saharan-africa (accessed 14 June 2012).

[8]   Hall V, Reimar W T, Ole H, Nicolai L: Diabetes in Sub Saharan Africa 1999-2011: Epi-
      demiology and public health implications. a systematic review. BMC Public Health
      2011, 11:564.

[9]   Ik Yong Kim. Gangrene: The Prognostic Factors and Validation of Severity Index in
      Fournier's Gangrene. Current Concepts and Management Options, Alexander Vitin
      (Ed.), ISBN: 978-953-307-386-6, InTech, Available from: http://www.zums.ac.ir/files/
      research/site/medical/Surgery/Gangrene_Current_Concepts_and_Manage-
      ment_Options.pdf (accessed 20 December 2012).

[10] Ndubuisi Eke and John E. Raphael. Fournier's Gangrene. Current Concepts and
      Management Options, Alexander Vitin (Ed.), ISBN: 978-953-307-386-6, InTech, Avail-
      able   from: http://www.zums.ac.ir/files/research/site/medical/Surgery/
      Gangrene_Current_Concepts_and_Management_Options.pdf (accessed 20th Decem-
      ber 2012).

[11] Obalum, D.C & Okeke, GC. (2009). Lower limb amputations at a Nigerian private
      tertiary hospital. West Afr J Med. Jan;24-27.

[12] Vamos EP, Bottle A, Edmonds ME, Valabhji J, Majeed A, Millett C. Changes in the
      incidence of lower extremity amputations in individuals with and without diabetes
      in England between 2004 and 2008. Diabetes Care. 2010, 33(12):2592-7.

[13] Unuigbe EI, Ikhidero J, Ogbemudia AO, Bafor A, Isah AO. Multiple digital gangrene
      arising from traditional therapy: a case report. West Afr J Med. 2009 Nov-Dec;28(6):
      397-9. Available at http://www.ncbi.nlm.nih.gov/pubmed/20939153. (accessed 1 Oc-
      tober, 2012).

[14] Vivek Srivastava, Vaibhav Pandey and Somprakas Basu (2011). Intestinal Ischemia
      and Gangrene, Gangrene - Current Concepts and Management Options, Alexander
      Vitin (Ed.), ISBN: 978-953-307-386-6, InTech, Available from: http://www.intechop-
      en.com/books/gangrene-current-concepts-and-management-options/intestinal-ische-
      mia-and-gangrene (accessed 28 September 2012).

Chapter 3

Trends in Amputation

F. Santosa and K. Kröger

Additional information is available at the end of the chapter

1. Introduction

Representatives of government health departments and patients' organisations from all European countries met with diabetes experts under the aegis of WHO Regional Offices for Europe and the International Diabetes Federation (IDF), European region, in St Vincent, Italy on 10–12 October 1989. Within this declaration of the five-year targets was to reduce by one half the rates of limb amputations for diabetic gangrene.

There is an ongoing discussion whether this target could be achieved. In the recent years some data were published presenting promising numbers of decreasing amputation rates.

2. United States

Rowe et al. analysed data from a Nationwide Inpatient Sample (NIS) from 1996-2005 in the United States (Rowe et al. 2009). The NIS included 74 millions discharge records and was used as source data regarding treatment patterns for patients with PAD. Since 1988, the NIS has constructed a dataset comprising approximately 20% of the hospital discharges within the United States. In order to develop a sample that most accurately represents the total universe of domestic hospitalizations, hospitals are sampled according to specific characteristics (strata), including geographic region, hospital ownership, urban/rural location, and teaching status. Each discharge in the NIS dataset, therefore represents approximately five domestic discharges. This 5:1 ratio is not constant across the NIS sample, however. Certain combinations of strata may be under-sampled or over-sampled due to pragmatic considerations of sampling design. When this occurs, the importance (weight) assigned to a specific hospitalization may be greater or less than five. Unless specifically stated, all data and analyses in this study are reported using the weighting scheme included with the NIS.

Average annual admissions receiving major amputation in the years 1996 to 2005 were 41,275. 53.2% were females. Individuals undergoing major amputation were older (72.2 years) than those that had open or endovascular procedures performed. The number of major amputations fell significantly between 1996 and 2005, by an estimated 6.4% per year (P <0.05) (Fig 1). Rates of decrease were more dramatic in the above 75 age group than in the younger age groups.

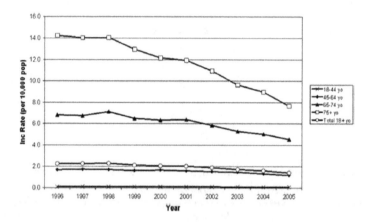

Figure 1. Rates of major amputation for peripheral arterial disease by age in the United States from 1996 to 2005. Overall incidence rate reflects population-adjusted incidence rate among individuals aged 18years and older in the United States (adjusted to 1996 population). (Rowe et al., 2009)

The authors also analyzed population-based rates of major amputation by diagnosis (PAD, non-atheroslerotic PVD, infection, malignancy, trauma, and other/unspecified). The vast majority of the reduction in population-based rates of major lower extremity amputations is due to decreases in amputation rates for PAD (Fig. 2).

A more recent publication from Li et al. based on the same population analysed the period from 1988 to 2008. The age-adjusted nontraumatic lower-extremity amputation per 1,000 persons among those diagnosed with diabetes and aged ≥40 years decreased from 11.2 in 1996 to 3.9 in 2008 (absolute percent -8.6%; P < 0.01), while rates among persons without diagnosed diabetes changed little. (Li et al., 2012)

In 2009 Goodney et al. published data based on the Medicare population (Goodney et al., 2009). The Medicare population included all people 65 years and older and regardless of age, every citizen with a recognized disability and each citizen with acute renal failure, which makes long-term dialysis or a kidney transplant needed. All Medicare claims from the Centers for Medicare and Medicaid Services between 1996 and 2006, using the Medicare Physician/ Supplier Procedure Summary Master File were included. This is a 100% sample of all Part B claims from all insurance carriers. Codes including a 250 modifier represented a procedure done on both sides of the body; therefore, any code with this modifier was multiplied by two in order to account for each limb. The absolute size of the Medicare population remained was rather stable over the study period, (31.7 million beneficiaries in 1996, 31.9 million beneficiaries in 2006). Presented were only unadjusted data reported per 100,000 beneficiaries. Rates of major amputations, defined as above-knee or below-knee amputation, coded according to current procedural terminology were examined over the study period. Given that lesser amputations at the metatarsal or single toe level are not generally considered failures of limb salvage, amputations at lesser levels were not included in this analysis. To allow for comparison over time, annual rates were again normalized to reflect incidence rates per 100,000 Medicare beneficiaries, and RRs were calculated similarly as above. The author assumed that the proportion of major lower extremity amputation due to peripheral vascular disease remained constant over the study period, as prior analyses have demonstrated that fewer than 15% of major lower extremity amputations are traumatic in nature, and little change has occurred in the incidence of traumatic amputation in recent years.

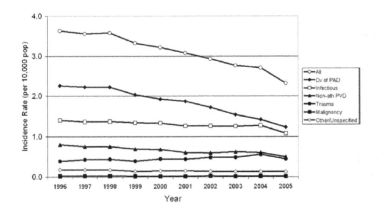

Figure 2. Rates of major amputation by indication in the United States from 1996 to 2005. Incidence rates are population-adjusted to 1996. (Rowe et al., 2009)

A distinct decline in the population based rates of major lower extremity amputation occurred between 1996 and 2006 (Fig. 3)). Overall, the rate of below and above-knee amputation decreased from 263 to 188 amputations per 100,000 Medicare beneficiaries, a 29% decline (RR 0.71, 95% CI 0.6-0.8). This decline began in 2000, and remains progressive throughout the next 6 years. Results were not different if above-knee amputations were studied distinctly from below-knee amputations as both decreased in similar magnitude.

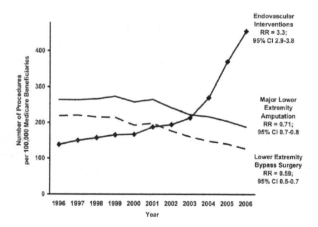

Figure 3. Trends in endovascular interventions, major amputation, and lower extremity bypass surgery, 1996-2006. *RR,* Risk ratio; *CI,* confidence interval. (Goodney et al., 2009)

3. Australia

In contrast to the data from the United States the number of diabetes-related hospitalisations for major lower limb amputation did not show a significant trend in Far North Queensland, Australia. (O'Rouke et al. 2012). There was a discrepancy of 6 (3.7%) in 161 cases over 10 years from 1998-99 to 2007-08. The number of diabetes-related hospitalisations for major lower limb amputation did not show a significant trend during this period, with an annual percentage change of -0.32% (P=0.915). Thus, there was a modest reduction in the hospitalisation rate for major lower limb amputation over the 10-year period only, demonstrating the need for improvements in the organisation of care.

4. United Kingdom

Recent data from the United Kingdom are in line with the findings from Australia. Vamos et al identified all patients aged >16 years who underwent any nontraumatic amputation in England between 2004 and 2008 using national hospital activity data from all National Health Service hospitals. During the study period the incidence of diabetes-related amputations decreased by 9.1%, from 27.5 to 25.0 per 10,000 people with diabetes (p>0.2) (Fig. 4). The incidence of minor and major amputations did not significantly change (15.7-14.9 and 11.8-10.2 per 10,000 people with diabetes; p=0.66 and p=0.29, respectively). Poisson regression analysis showed no statistically significant change in diabetes-related amputation incidence over time (0.98 decrease per year [95% CI 0.93-1.02]; p=0.12) (Vamos et a. 2010).

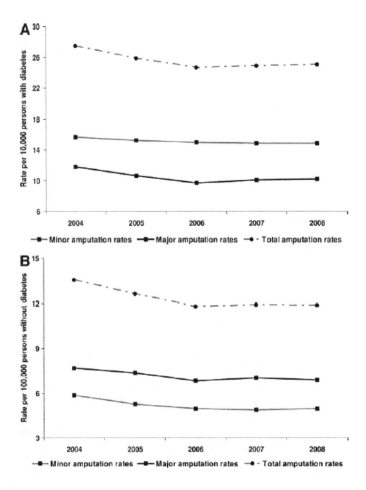

Figure 4. Changes in minor and major amputation incidence rates in (A) individuals with diabetes expressed per 10,000 people with diabetes and (B) individuals without diabetes expressed per 100,000 people without diabetes. (Vamos et al. 2010)

Incidence of lower extremity amputations was significantly higher among men than among women with diabetes (P < 0.001). However, changes in overall lower extremity amputations rates did not significantly differ between men and women (19.9 to 18.3 vs. 7.6 to 6.7 per 10,000 people with diabetes; P = 0.81). When stratified by age, the incidence was the highest among individuals aged ≥65 years in both men and women. Poisson regression analysis showed no significant decrease in incidence of amputations after adjustment for age, sex, year, and level of amputation (0.98 decrease per year [95% CI 0.93–1.02]; P = 0.12).

The number of people without diabetes who underwent a lower extremity amputations decreased during the study period. Although the percentage of men undergoing minor amputations increased significantly, male predominance was not evident among minor amputees. Amputation incidence (minor and major combined) decreased from 13.6 per 100,000 people without diabetes in 2004 to 11.9 per 100,000 people without diabetes in 2008.

Incidence of minor lower extremity amputations decreased significantly from 5.9 to 5.0 per 100,000 people without diabetes (P < 0.01). There was a nonsignificant reduction in the incidence of major lower extremity amputations among individuals without diabetes, from 7.7 to 6.9 per 100,000 people (P = 0.39) (Fig. 1).

The fall in lower extremity amputations rates was achieved between 2004 and 2006, and incidence rates remained constant afterward for both minor and major procedures. Incidence of lower extremity amputations declined among both men and women.

Poisson regression analysis showed that the decline in nondiabetes-related lower extremity amputations was marginally significant after adjustment for age, sex, level of amputation, and year (0.97 decrease by year [95% CI 0.93–1.00], P= 0.059).

5. Spain

A Spanish analysis did not report a decrease in the incidence of lower limb amputation in Andalusia from 1998 to 2006 in the population with and without diabetes (Almaraz et al., 2012). Andalusia, one of the 17th Spanish Autonomous Communities in Spain, had a total population of 7,975,672 inhabitants in 2006. The Andalusian Health Service, guarantees health care to almost 100% of the population (free, universal care). The information system is the same for the whole of Andalusia and all main diagnosis from people admitted to hospital are recorded in the CMBD (Conjunto Mı́nimo Ba´ sico de Datos, a basic set of data), at patient discharge. This data collection (CMBD) is mandatory and this collection of data with a standardized methodology was introduced in Spain in 1982. These data are registered in accordance with the ICD-9-CM, and then send them to the Andalusian Health Service Central Services.

During the study period 1998–2006 a total of 16,210 lower limb amputations were performed in people aged ≥30 years old in Andalusia. Of these, 11,770 (72.6%) were in patients with diabetes mellitus and 4440 (27.4%) in individuals without diabetes mellitus. The average age of patients who underwent lower limb amputations was (mean ± SD): 70.6 ± 11.6 years; patients with diabetes mellitus were aged 70.3 ± 10.7 years and patients without diabetes mellitus were 71.3 ± 13.7 years old (p <0.05). In the population with diabetes the standardized incidence of all lower limb amputation was found to be 34.0 per 10,000 (95% CI, 31.5-37.2) in 2004-2006. There was an estimated incidence increase for all lower limb amputation by 14% and for minor lower limb amputation by 13.6% in 2004-2006. In people with diabetes the RR increased by 31.6% as compared to the first period (Fig. 5).

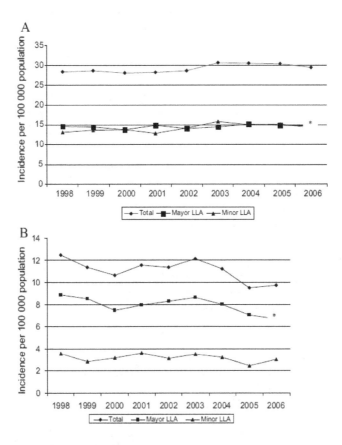

Figure 5. Changes in total, major and minor LLA incidence rates in patients with diabetes mellitus (A) and without diabetes mellitus (B) expressed per 100,000 inhabitants. *p < 0.05 (Poisson regression analysis).(Almaraz et al. 2012)

6. Germany

In 2011 Moysidis et al published data from Germany based on the national statistics (DRG statistics) provided from the Federal Statistical Office. The DRG-statistics include data from all hospitals in Germany that use the DRG system, which are more than 99 %. These hospitals are legally obliged to deliver extensive data on hospital treatment, including demographic data, diagnoses, co-morbidities, complications, and procedures to the "Institute for the Hospital Remuneration System" which uses the data for a yearly adaptation of the German DRG system and transmits them to the Federal Statistical Office.

Major amputation

		total	< 50	50-60	60-70	70-80	"/>80
all							
	2005	23.3	1	14	43	94	181
	2006	22.6	1	14	41	87	173
	2007	21.8	1	14	37	85	161
	2008	21.0	1	13	36	79	153
Males							
	2005	27.0	1	22	67	135	216
	2006	26.6	1	23	65	125	208
	2007	25.6	2	22	59	124	180
	2008	25.1	1	21	58	116	178
Females							
	2005	19.7	1	5	20	63	168
	2006	18.7	1	6	18	57	158
	2007	18.2	1	6	16	54	152
	2008	17.1	1	5	16	49	142

Minor amputation

		total	< 50	50-60	60-70	70-80	"/>80
all							
	2005	35.0	3	31	79	144	183
	2006	36.1	3	33	81	147	180
	2007	36.6	3	33	78	148	180
	2008	38.1	3	33	80	148	192
Males							
	2005	47.4	4	51	129	224	266
	2006	49.5	4	54	133	230	259
	2007	50.6	4	54	129	234	261
	2008	53.7	4	55	134	240	285
Females							
	2005	23.1	2	12	31	83	150
	2006	23.1	1	11	32	82	148
	2007	23.1	2	12	29	80	146
	2008	23.2	2	11	29	76	151

Table 1. Age-adjusted incidence of major (OPS 5 – 864) and minor (OPS 5 – 865) amputations per 100.000 inhabitants in Germany from 2005 to 2008 excluding those patients amputated for injury and toxicity, musculoskeletal disorder, diseases of skin and subcutaneous tissue and malignant neoplasm. (Moysidis et al. 2011)

The total number of patients hospitalised with the principal diagnosis peripheral arterial disease and neurovascular disease increased from 163,520 in 2005 to 178,086 in 2008. Within the same time period the total number of major amputations decreased from 25,315 in 2005 to 23,009 in 2008 whilst the number of minor amputations increased form 37,690 in 2005 to 40,276 in 2008. After age adjustment major amputation rates still decreased for both genders (Tab. 1) Overall minor amputation rates do not show such a decrease but increased in males and remained unchanged in females.

7. Discussion

All in all there is a great variation in the incidence of lower extremity amputations, even within one country. In England the incidences of amputations in adults determined from hospital episode statistics over 3 years to 31 March 2010 showed large variation between 151 Primary Care Trusts. Incidence varied eightfold across Primary Care Trusts in people both with diabetes (range 0.64-5.25 per 1,000 person-years) and without (0.03-0.24 per 1,000 person-years). Amputations in people with diabetes varied tenfold-both major (range 0.22-2.20 per 1,000 person-years) and minor (range 0.30-3.25 per 1,000 person-years). (Holman et al. 2012).

Moxey et al. performed an electronic search using the EMBASE and MEDLINE databases from 1989 until 2010 for incidence of lower extremity amputation. There reviewed showed significant global variation exists in the incidence of lower extremity amputation. Incidence of all forms of lower extremity amputation ranges from 46.1 to 9600 per 100.000 in the population with diabetes compared with 5.8-31 per 100.000 in the total population. Major amputation ranges from 5.6 to 600 per 100.000 in the population with diabetes and from 3.6 to 68.4 per 100.000 in the total population (Moxey et al., 2011). The authors mad the following conclusions:

- Significant reductions in incidence of lower extremity amputation have been shown in specific at-risk populations after the introduction of specialist diabetic foot clinics.

- Ethnicity and social deprivation play a significant role but it is the role of diabetes and its complications that is most profound.

- Lower extremity amputation reporting methods demonstrate significant variation with no single standard upon which to benchmark care.

Thus, all data and the specific conclusion drawn from these data, respectively, have to be handled with care as there are no lower extremity amputation reporting standards used that would allow benchmark (Moxey et al., 2011). Especially data regarding minor amputation rates can be assumed to underestimate the truth. An unknown but probably high number of patients suffering from foot lesion is effectively treated in outdoor settings and do not appear in the analysed data basis. In light of the rising prevalence of diabetes mellitus minor amputations might mirror the burden of the problem more accurately, whereas major amputation rates might give an insight in effectiveness of treatment strategies. Minor amputation rates that do not decrease or even increase show that prevention of foot lesions is not effectively achieved. Decreasing major amputations rates show, that if patients will get optimal treatment this treatment is able to prevent deterioration of the lesion in some patients.

Author details

F. Santosa[1] and K. Kröger[2]
1 Klinik Angiologi & Kardiologi "Waringin Medika", Jakarta, Indonesia
2 Department of Angiology, HELIOS Klinikum Krefeld, Germany

References

[1] Goodney P.P., Beck A.W., Nagle J., Welch H.G., Zwolak R.M., 2009. National trends in lower extremity bypass surgery, endovascular interventions, and major amputations. J. Vasc. Surg. 50,54-60.

[2] Gutacker N, Neumann A, Santosa F, Moysidis T, Kröger K. Amputations in PAD patients: data from the German Federal Statistical Office. Vasc Med. 2010;15:9-14

[3] Rowe V.L., Lee W., Weaver F.A., Etzioni D., 2009. Patterns of treatment for peripheral arterial disease in the United States: 1996-2005. J. Vasc. Surg. 49, 910-917.

[4] Almaraz MC, González-Romero S, Bravo M, Caballero FF, Palomo MJ, Vallejo R, Esteva I, Calleja F, Soriguer F. Incidence of lower limb amputations in individuals with and without diabetes mellitus in Andalusia (Spain) from 1998 to 2006. Diabetes Res Clin Pract. 2012;95:399-405.

[5] Li Y, Burrows NR, Gregg EW, Albright A, Geiss LS. Declining rates of hospitalization for nontraumatic lower-extremity amputation in the diabetic population aged 40 years or older: U.S., 1988-2008. Diabetes Care. 2012;35:273-277.

[6] O'Rourke SR, Steffen CM, Raulli A, Tulip FJ. Diabetes-related major lower limb amputation in Far North Queensland, 1998-2008. Aust Health Rev. 2012 Mar;36(1):105-9.

[7] Vamos EP, Bottle A, Edmonds ME, Valabhji J, Majeed A, Millett C. Changes in the incidence of lower extremity amputations in individuals with and without diabetes in England between 2004 and 2008. Diabetes Care. 2010;33:2592-2597

[8] Moxey PW, Gogalniceanu P, Hinchliffe RJ, Loftus IM, Jones KJ, Thompson MM, Holt PJ. Lower extremity amputations--a review of global variability in incidence. Diabet Med. 2011;28:1144-1153.

[9] Holman N, Young RJ, Jeffcoate WJ. Variation in the recorded incidence of amputation of the lower limb in England. Diabetologia. 2012 Mar 8. [Epub ahead of print]

[10] Moysidis T, Nowack T, Eickmeyer F, Waldhausen P, Brunken A, Hochlenert D, Engels G, Santosa F, Luther B, Kröger K. Trends in amputations in people with hospital admissions for peripheral arterial disease in Germany. Vasa. 2011;40:289-295.

Chapter 4

Perineal Gas Gangrene: Two Cases Report and Review of the Literature

Slim Jarboui, Abdelwaheb Hlel, Alifa Daghfous and
Lamia Rezgui Marhoul

Additional information is available at the end of the chapter

1. Introduction

Gas gangrene or clostridialmyonecrosis is a necrotic infection of skin and soft tissue and it is characterized by the presence of gas under the skin which is produced by clostridium. It is a potentially lethal disease which spreads quickly in soft tissues of the body.

Tissue necrosis id due to production of exotoxins by spore forming gas producing bacteria in an environment of low oxygen.

Herein we report two cases of perineal gas gangrene which were treated early with surgical debridement, antibiotics and hyperbaroxygenotherapy. Additionally, a review of the literature regarding gas gangrene is presented.

2. Case n°1

A 57 –year-old male presented to the emergency department reporting three days of worsening perineal and scrotal pain and swelling. He denied diabetes or trauma. His genitourinary examination revealed a draining lesion in his left inguinal region with surrounding indurations and cellulites extending onto his scrotum. His perineum was edematous and tender with a distinct region of ecchymosis and crepitus. The patient's blood pressure was 100/56 mmhg; his body temperature rose to 39°C. The laboratory data demonstrated severe infection with white blood cell count of 27000/mm3, a C-reactive protein level of 158mg/dl and a blood sugar level of 14,09mmom/L. Computed tomography showed a perineal collection extended to the left ischio rectal region with emphysematous gangrene extended to the pelvis among the left iliac muscle and to the left inguinal region (Fig. 1). These results con-firmed a diagnosis of gas gangrene of the perineum due to ischio rectal abscess. Shortly after arrival, the patient was transferred to the operating room for surgical debridement (Fig.2) with broad spectrum antibiotics (intravenous ampicillin-Sulbactam and metronidazole). Blood cultures were negative, and Gram stain of pus and necrotic tissue showed Gram posi-tive rods, which were later confirmed as C. Perfingens. The patient was also treated with hy-perbaric oxygen therapy postoperatively. We began HBOT five days after surgical debridement. He was exposed to pure oxygen at 2, 5 atmospheres absolute pressure for 100 to 120 min. This procedure was repeated three times weekly for one month.He had an un-eventful recovery and was discharged after 15 days of hospitalization.

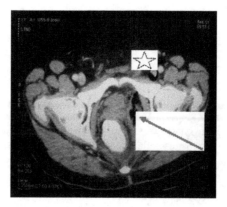

Figure 1. Computed tomography showed a perineal collection extended to the left ischio rectal region (red Arrow) with emphysematous gangrene extended to the pelvis among the left iliac muscle and to the left inguinal region (As-terix)

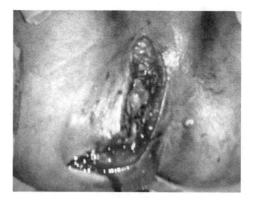

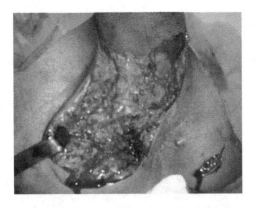

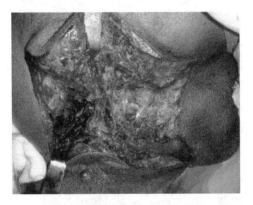

Figure 2. Perineal gangrene: Aggressive approach with extended surgical excision.

3. Case n°2

A 45-year-male was admitted with a three-day history of persistent perineal pain after initial intervention for anal abscess. There was no medical history of diabetes or others abnormalities.On examination, he was normotensive, tachycardic, and pyrexial at 39, 4°C. Cardiovascular, respiratory and neurological examinations were no contributory. Abdominal examination revealed a non tender abdomen with no sign of peritonism. A balloon-like induration with retract-pain was found in the perineum and extended to the left scrotum with redness of the skin. Manual rectal examination demonstrated a very tender rectum. Blood tests revealed a slightly elevated white blood cell count of 11700/mm3, a C-reactive protein level of 118mg/dl and serum glucose was normal. A CT pelvis demonstrated collection in the bilateral ischio-rectal fossa, with gas in the perirectal region extended to the high pelvis

(Fig.3). Theses appearances were consistent with those of gas gangrene. The patient was commenced on IV benzylpznicillin, metronidazole with aggressive fluid resuscitation and was immediately subjected to wide debridement, necrotic tissues excision. Examination of the rectum revealed bilateral ischiorectal abscess, which were drained and necessitated a temporary diverting colostomy. Culture of tissue specimens obtained intraopeartively was negative. Postoperatively he remained septicaemic, inotrope dependent, and ventilated for the next three days. Daily surgical debridement with resection of additional necrotic tissue was performed with two times performed in the operating room under general anesthesia.. Over the next 8 days, he gradually improved, and weaned off the inotropes. Treatment was continued with tazocillin-metronidazone for two weeks. Additionally, hyperbaric oxygen therapy was performed starting two weeks after the operation for three weeks. We performed the same protocol like the first case reported. He was discharged from the hospital on postoperative day 40 with satisfactory and progressive healing of the injured wound. The patient successfully recovered within three months after the initial operation.

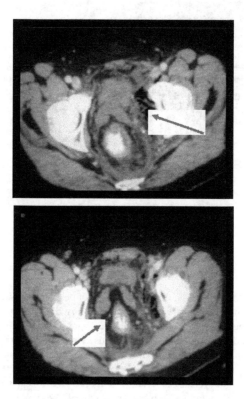

Figure 3. CT pelvis demonstrated collection in the bilateral ischio-rectal fossa, with gas in the perirectal region extended to the high pelvis

4. Discussion

Gas gangrene and perineal necrotizing fasciitis or Fournier's gangrene are rare but serious infections with acute onset, rapid progression, systemic toxemia and a high mortality rate [1,2]. It is defined as a synergistic, polymicrobial necrotizing fasciitis of the perineal, perirectal or genital area. The bacterial synergism of aerobic and anaerobic organisms, indigenous commensal below the pelvic diaphragm, results in the production of exotoxins that lead to tissue necrosis and the synthesis of insoluble substances gases that give rise to the characteristic, though not constant, subcutaneous emphysema of perineal gas gangrene or Fournier gangrene [1-5].

It is well known that usual causative organisms in gas gangrene are clostridial species. However, a variety of other organisms: coliforms, anaerobic streptococci, and bacteriodes may also produceinfection in which gas is demonstrable. Fermentation of glucose in tissues is thought to be the source of the gas in gangrenous infections.

The most common predisposing factors are diabetes mellitus and alcohol abuse [1,5-9].In a review of 1726 cases, published in the literature, diabetes mellitus was a factor in 20%[1]. Others important predisposing factors include in dwelling catheters, localized trauma, surgical procedure,ma-lignancy, steroids, chemotherapy and human immunodeficiency virus [9-13].

Nowadays, the cause of this perineal gangrene is usually identified, with only 10% of cases being idiopathic. The necrotizing process commonly originates with an infection in the ano-rectum, the urogenital tract, or the skin. The disease is most often due to a local infection adjacent to a point of entry, including abscess (particularly in the perineal, perirectal, and ischio rectal regions), anal fissures and colonic perforations [1, 5, 7, 14, 15]. It has also been reported secondary to rectal carcinoma and diverticulitis. The urologic forms include urethral strictures, chronic urinary tract infection, and epididimitis. Insect bites, burns, trauma, and circoncision, have been reported as causes of pediatric Fournier gangrene, which is rarely seen [14].

Pain is a common presenting complaint and may be the first sign in patients with gas gangrene. Bullae and the bluish skin discoloration are classic findings. Edema and crepitus are usually present at the time of diagnosis. The triad of pain, tachycardia out of proportion to fever and crepitus is highly suggestive of clostridialmyonecrosis. Crepitus is identified at physical examination in 19 -64% [14]. Soft-tissue gas may be present prior to the detection of clinical crepitus.Fournier gangrene is classically associated with ecchymotic changes, edema, erythamatous and drainage from wounds.Systemic findings may include leukocytosis, dehydratation, tachycardia, thrombocytopenia, anemia, and hyperglycemia [3, 6, 14, 15].

Perineal gas gangrene tends to be polymicrobial in nature, with synergy of aerobic and anaerobic bacteria. The most commonly found bacteria are Escherichia Coli, followed by Bacteriodes and Streptococcal species. Other bacteria involved include Staphylococcus, Enterococcus, Clostridium, Pseudomonas, Klebsiella and proteus species [1, 8, 10, 14].

Infection in perineal gas gangrene tends to spread along the fascial plans. Infection arising from the anal triangle can spread along the Colles fascia (superficial perineal fascia) and progress anteriorly along the Dartos fascia to involve the scrotum and penis. It can pass also superiorly along the Scarpa fascia to involve the anterior abdominal wall. If the Colles fascia is interrupted, the infection can spread to the ischiorectal fossa and subsequently to the buttocks and thighs [14].

Although the diagnosis of gas gangrene is often made clinically, emergency computed tomography (CT) can lead to early diagnosis with accurate assessment of disease extent. CT not only helps evaluate the perineal structures that become involved by gangrene, but also helps assess the retroperitoneum; to which the disease can spread[14,15]. Findings at CT include asymetric-fascialthickening, subcutaneous emphysema, fluid collections, and abscess formation. Subcutaneous emphysema is the hallmark of gas gangrene but is not seen in all cases.

Initial plain film may show moderate –to - large amounts of soft tissue gas. At radiography, hyperleucencies representing soft tissue gas may be seen in the region overlying the scrotum and perineum. Radiographic evidence of soft tissue gas may be present before clinical crepitus is detected, and its absence at physical examination should not exclude the diagnosis of Fournier gangrene. Ultrasonography (US) can be used to detect fluid or gas within the soft tissue. The thickened scrotal wall contains hyperchoic foci that demonstrate reverberation artifact[14-17].

CT imaging can detect smaller amounts of soft tissue gas than plain radiographs and can demonstrate fluid collections that track along the deep fascial planes. It often demonstrate the underlying cause of Fournier gangrenesuch as perineal abscesses, fistulous tracts, incarcerated inguinal hernias, and sources of infection due to intra-abdominal and retroperitoneal processes.

The management included surgical debridement of the necrotic tissue with incisions and drainage of the involved areas, antibiotic therapy and surgical intensive care [1, 5, 8, 14-20]. Early diagnosis and aggressive management are essential as overwhelming sepsis may quickly develop and is associated with a significant mortality rate reported as 16% in the Meta analysis of Eke [1]. The Fournier's gangrene severity index (FGSI) score is a numeric score proposed by Laor et al in 1995 to prognosticate on the outcome of the disease [4, 10, 21-22]. It is obtained from a combination of admission physiologic parameters, including temperature, heart and respiration rates, sodium, potassium, creatinine, WBC counts, hematocrit, and sodium bicarbonates. It has been proposed that a FGSI score> 9indicates a 75% probability of mortality and score < 9 is associated with a 78% probability of survival [21].

The radical removal of all necrotic tissue at the first operation is crucial to the survival of the patient. A second look operation should be performed at 24-48 hours to ensure that all necrotic tissue has been cleared. Multiple debridements may be necessary to remove all nonviable tissue.Patients with incomplete drainage and debridement or who undergo treatment with antibiotics alone have a poor prognosis [1, 18, 21, 22].

Antibiotic choice is variable and may be institutionally dependent. Prompt initiation of antimicrobial treatment covering arobic and anaeorobic organism is critical. Ampicillin-sulbactam or piperacillin-tazobactam or ticarcillin-clavulateare suggested empiric regimens, whereas antibiotic treatment should be tailored according to the susceptibility results. Neutralization of clostridial or streptococcal circulating toxins by the use of intravenous immune globulin has shown promising results but there are no data to support strong recommendations for its regular use in patients with gas gangrene [6].

Some authors have demonstrated that sugars (sucrose, glucose) inhibited the production of the main protein toxin (alpha toxin, theta toxin), responsible for the onset and progression of gas gangrene [23].

Adjunctive hyperbaric oxygen therapy (HBOT) has been shown to increase survival in animal model and in humans, to suppress alpha toxin of clostridium, enhance leukocyte-killing activity, enhance destruction of anaerobic bacteria and improve tissue repair in poorly vascularized tissues [1,18,24,25]. HBOT has shown some promise in shortening hospital stay, increasing wound healing, and decreasing the gangrenous spread in conjunction with surgical debridement and antibiotics. It may decrease the number of debridement required. It increases tissue oxygen issue tension to a high level that in turn inhibits and kills anaerobic bacteria while suppressing aerobic bacteria proliferation [6,14, 24, 25].

After healthy granulation has appeared, the healing time can be shortened with reconstructive procedures.

5. Conclusion

Gas gangrene of the genitalia and perineum continues to be a diagnostic and therapeutic challenge. Physician and emergency medicine personnel should always maintain high index of suspicion of this severe infection even in the absence of diabetes or others co morbidities and predisposing factors. CT scan defines the extent of the disease and is of greatest benefit in planning the surgical debridement. Early diagnosis and complete surgical debridement of all necrosis tissue are the most important prognostic factors. In addition, we may also consider consulting for HBOT and intensive care if appropriate.

Computed tomography showed a perineal collection extended to the left ischio rectal region (red Arrow) with emphysematous gangrene extended to the pelvis among the left iliac muscle and to the left inguinal region (Asterix)

Author details

Slim Jarboui[1*], Abdelwaheb Hlel[1], Alifa Daghfous[2] and Lamia Rezgui Marhoul[2]

*Address all correspondence to: drslimjarboui@yahoo.fr

1 Faculté de Medecine de Sousse, Department of General Surgery- Hospital of SidiBouzid, University of Medicine of Sousse, Tunisia

2 Faculté de Medecine de Sousse, Department of Radiology- Trauma Center of Ben Arous, University of Medicine of Sousse, Tunisia

References

[1]   Eke N. Fournier's Gangrene: a review of 1726 cases. Br J Surg 2000; 87:718-728.

[2]   Mercer, N., Davies, D. M., & Gas, Gangrene. B. M. J.

[3]   Lehner, P. J., Powell, H., & Gas, Gangrene. Overwhelming infection responsive to surgical and medical treatment. BMJ; 303: 2406242.

[4]   Wolf Chelsea T, Wolf Stephen J. Fournier Gangrene. Western Journal of Emergency Medicine 2010; 11: 101-102.

[5]   Paty, R., & Smith, A. D. Gangrene and Fournier's gangrene. UrolClin North Am (1992). , 149-62.

[6]   Aggelidakis, J., Lasithiotakis, K., Topalidou, A., Koutroumpas, J., Kouvidis, G., & Katonis, P. Limb Salvage after gas gangrene: a case report and review of the literature. World Journal of Emergency Surgery (2011).

[7]   Cabrera, H., Skoczdopole, L., Marini, M., Della Giovanna, P., Saponaro, A., & Echeverria, C. Necrotizing gangrene of the genitalia and perineum. Int J Dermatol (2002). , 41, 847-51.

[8]   Ghosh, S., Bal, Abhijit. M., Malik, I., & Collier, A. Fatal Morganellamorganiibacteraemia in a diabetic patient with gas gangrene. Journal of medical Microbiology (2009). , 58, 965-967.

[9]   Tanaka S, Fuji S, Ohashi M, Yamamoto M, Sek J, Wada M. A Survival case of diabetes with nonclostridial Gas Gangrene. Jap J Med 1983; 22; 40-44.

[10] Youda, J., Honma, R., Yahagin, T., & Omoto, E. Fournier's Gangrene in a patient receiving treatment for Idiopathic Thrombocytopenic Purpura. Inter Med (2011). , 50, 2019-2011.

[11] Yoshida N, Yamazaki S, Takayama T. A Case of Fournier's Gangrene after liver transplantation: BioScience Trends 2011; 5: 223-225.

[12] Kiel N, Ho V, Pascoe A. A Case of gas gangrene in an immunosuppressed crohn's patient. World J Gastroenterol 2011; 17: 3856-58.

[13] Cooney, D. R., & Cooney, N. L. Gas Gangrene and osteomyelitis of the foot in a diabetic patient treated with tea tree oil. International Journal of Emergency Medicine. (2011).

[14] Cullen, I. M., Larkin, J. O., Moore, M., Fitzerald, E., O', Riordan. M., & Rogers, E. Fournier's Gangrene _Findings on Computed Tomography. Case study The Scientific World Journal (2007). , 7, 1839-1841.

[15] Levenson Robin B, Singh Ajay K, Novelline Robert A. Fournier Gangrene: Role of Imaging. Radiographics 2008; 28: 519-528.

[16] Tsait, M. J., Lient, C. T., Chang, W. A., Weit, P. J., Hsieh, M. H., Tsait, Y. M., et al., & Transperineal, . TransperinealUlsonography in the diagnosis of Fournier's gangrene. Ultrasound ObstetGynecol (2010). , 36, 387-391.

[17] Uppot R.N, Levy H.M, Patel PH. Case 54: Fournier gangrene.Radiology(2003). , 226, 115-117.

[18] Korhonen, K., Klossner, J., & Niinikoski, J. Management of clostridial gas gangrene and the role of hyperbaric oxygen. Ann ChirGynacol (1999). , 88, 139-42.

[19] Freischlag, J. A., Ajalat, G., & Busuttil, R. W. Treatment of necrotizing soft tissue infections. The need for a new approach. Am J Surg (1985). , 149, 751-5.

[20] Hiro, M., & Niinikoski, J. Management of perineal necrotizing fasciitis (Fournier's Gangrene). Ann ChirGynaecol (1989). , 78, 277-81.

[21] Tovat, J. R., Cordoba, L., & Devesa, J. M. Prognostic factors in Fournier gangrene. Asian Journal of Surgery (2012). , 35, 37-41.

[22] Eke N. Fournier4s gangrene, still an enigma. J Postgrad Med 2008; 54:83-4.

[23] Mendez, M. B., Goni, A., Ramirez, W., & Grau, R. R. Sugar inhibits the production of the toxins that trigger clostridial gas gangrene. MicrobPathog. (2012). , 52, 85-91.

[24] Hirn, M. (1993). Hyperbaric oxygen in the treatment of gas gangrene and perineal necrotizing fasciitis. A clinical and experimental study. Eur J SurgSupp.

[25] Korhonen, K. Hyperbaric oxygen therapy in acute necrotizing infections with a special reference to the effects on tissue gas tensions. Ann ChirGynaecolSupp (2000). ; ., 214, 7-36.

Chapter 5

Diabetic Foot Ulcer

Bardia Farzamfar, Reza Nazari and
Saeed Bayanolhagh

Additional information is available at the end of the chapter

1. Introduction

Every emergency physician has seen diabetic foot ulcers in their nascent stage, at a stage requiring minimal treatment with good follow-up, when they require aggressive treatment, and at a stage when amputation is a foregone conclusion. Ulcerations of the foot in diabetics are common; most diabetics will get them. Not only are they disabling, they also are limb- and life-threatening. [1]

It is estimated that approximately 15% of diabetic people world-wide will at some stage develop diabetic foot ulceration. The prevalence of active foot ulceration varies from approximately 1% in certain European and North American studies to more than 11% in reports from some African countries (table 1). Although there have been many developments in recent years which encourage optimism for future improvement in diabetic foot care, there is still much to be done; the recent data from the Netherlands show that with a concerted team approach, it is possible to increase the numbers of foot clinics with the provision of podiatry services by more than 100%. However, many countries still lack proper podiatry and specialist nursing provision and there remains much to be done in the next millennium to improve the lot of the diabetic patient with foot problems. [2,3] In general, in diabetic patients, the incidence of foot ulcers ranges from 1.0% to 4.1%, and the incidence of lower-extremity amputations ranges from 2.1 to 13.7 per 1000. [4-6]

The nerves of the leg and foot serve to propel the body through the actions of the legs, feet, and toes while maintaining balance, both while the body is moving and when it is at rest. Sensory nerves are of course present throughout the lower extremities; however, with the exception of the bottom of the foot, they play a lesser role here than in the upper extremities. Primarily, this section of the peripheral nervous system sends and receives signals regarding

Study (country)	Population base	N	Prevalence (%)	Annual incidence[a](%)	Ulcer definition	Ulcer ascertainment method
Rith-Najarian et al. (US)	Chippewa Indian residents with diabetes	266	-	0.6 (Non-neuropathic subjects)	Full thickness plantar foot lesion	Retrospective review of medical records/clinical examinations
Walters et al. (UK)	Registered patients with diabetes from 10 UK general practices	1077	2.9 (current) 7.4 (History of ulcer)	-	Wagner grade ≥1 foot lesion	Direct examination and structured interview
Moss et al. (US)	Population-based samples of persons with diabetes	1834	10.6 (History of ulcers at baseline)	2.2	???	Medical history questionnaire administered at baseline and 4 years later
Kumar et al. (UK)	Type 2 diabetes patients registered in three UK cities	811	1.4 (Current) 5.3 (History of ulcer)	-	Wagner grade ≥1 foot lesion	Direct exam by trained observers (current), and structured interview (history of ulcer)
Abbott et al. (UK)	Randomized controlled trial cohort	1035	-	3.6	Full-thickness lesion requiring hospital treatment	Direct examination at least every 13 weeks
Ramsey et al. (US)	Registered adult type 1 or 2 diabetes patients in a large HMO (1992-1995)	8905	-	1.9	ICD-codes: 707.1 (ulcer of lower leg)	Medical billing record audit
Abbott et al. (UK)	Registered type 1 and 2 diabetes patients in six UK districts	9710	1.7 (Current)	2.2	Wagner grade ≥1 foot lesion	Clinical examination (plus chart review)
Muller et al. (Netherland)	1993-1998 registered type 2 diabetes patients	3827 person-years	-	2.1	Full-thickness skin loss on the foot	Abstracted medical records
Centers for Disease Control and Prevention (US)	US BRFSS respondents with diabetes, 2000-2002[b]	NS	11.8 (History of ulcer)	-	Foot sore that did not heal for >4 weeks	Random-digit-dialed telephone interview

???, not specified.

[a] Incidence is annualized unless otherwise noted.

[b] BRFSS, Behavioral Risk Factor Surveillance Survey.

Table 1. Selected population-based studies estimating incidence and prevalence of diabetic foot ulcers (adapted from LeMaster and Reiber, 2006) [7]

locomotion of the body. Some of the impulses are sent from various parts of the brain and spinal cord; some come from sense organs located in the joints, ligaments, and tendons; and some come from the muscles themselves.

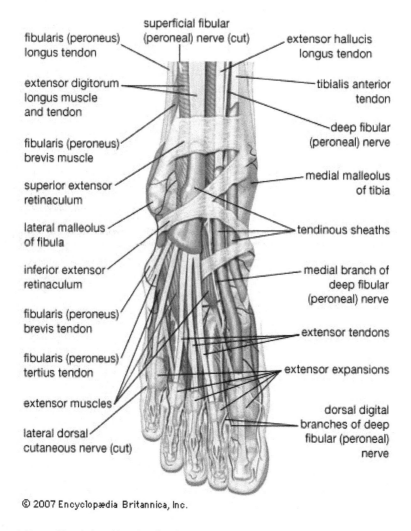

© 2007 Encyclopædia Britannica, Inc.

Figure 1. Nerves of foot. (adapted from Encyclopedia Britanica 2007)

The nerves of the leg and foot include the sacral plexus, lumbar plexus, femoral nerve, sciatic nerve, common fibular nerve, superficial fibular nerve, saphenous nerve, sural nerve, the deep and superficial peroneal nerves, and the tibial nerve (figure 1).

The nerves deliver messages to the brain that bring information about the angles and position of joints, the length and tension of muscles, or even the speed of movements so that through the interaction of the nervous system with the muscles of the lower extremities, balance may be maintained. The average nerve running from the base of the spine to the tip of a toe is about three feet long. This includes a major neural transmission network within the legs that produces contractions of groups of muscles and is responsible for larger muscular functions, such as running, walking or swimming. Finer nerve bundles command the many small bones of the toes to create the constant, subtle shifting of the feet that keeps us from falling down.

2. Peripheral neuropathy

Peripheral neuropathy is damage to nerves of the peripheral nervous system, which may be caused either by diseases of or trauma to the nerve or the side-effects of systemic illness.

The four cardinal patterns of peripheral neuropathy are polyneuropathy, mononeuropathy, mononeuritis multiplex and autonomic neuropathy. The most common form is (symmetrical) peripheral polyneuropathy, which mainly affects the feet and legs. The form of neuropathy may be further broken down by cause, or the size of predominant fiber involvement, i.e., large fiber or small fiber peripheral neuropathy. Frequently the cause of a neuropathy cannot be identified and it is designated as being idiopathic.

Neuropathy may be associated with varying combinations of weakness, autonomic changes, and sensory changes. Loss of muscle bulk or fasciculations, a particular fine twitching of muscle, may be seen. Sensory symptoms encompass loss of sensation and "positive" phenomena including pain. Symptoms depend on the type of nerves affected (motor, sensory, or autonomic) and where the nerves are located in the body. One or more types of nerves may be affected. Common symptoms associated with damage to the motor nerve are muscle weakness, cramps, and spasms. Loss of balance and coordination may also occur. Damage to the sensory nerve can produce tingling, numbness, and a burning pain. Pain associated with this nerve is described in various ways such as the following: burning, freezing, or electric-like, extreme sensitivity to touch. The autonomic nerve damage causes problems with involuntary functions leading to symptoms such as abnormal blood pressure and heart rate, reduced ability to perspire, constipation, bladder dysfunction (e.g., incontinence), and sexual dysfunction. [8-10]

3. Sensory neuropathy

Sensory neuropathy affects the nerves that carry messages from the skin, bones and muscles to the brain. As the name suggests, it tends to influence the senses, in particular touch, and affects how we feel temperature, pain and other sensations. It is the most common form of neuropathy, mainly occurring in nerves in the feet and legs, but can sometimes occur in the arms and hands. It can lead to a loss of feeling and a failure to sense pain. For example, if you trod on something sharp, stepped in to a hot bath or wore ill-fitting shoes, you may not be aware of damage to your feet. This lack of sensation can lead to damage becoming worse, and the potential for infection. Neuropathic ulcers may also occur. [11]

The symptoms of sensory neuropathy can include pain and numbness, tingling in the hands, legs or feet and extreme sensitivity to touch. Some treatments are available to help with the pain and tablets that are usually used for depression but can also have a calming effect on the nerves.

A test should be carried out at least every year, to check for signs of this type of neuropathy.

4. Motor neuropathy

Motor neuropathy affects the nerves that transmit signals to the muscles enabling them to carry out movements like walking and moving the hands. Sometimes painful, it causes muscle weakness and, in areas like the thigh, muscle wasting can occur. However it is possible for some people to recover from this condition after a period of time.

If the nerves that supply the small muscles in your feet are affected, motor neuropathy can lead to the development of foot deformities and alteration in the pressure distribution with walking or activity. Wasting of these muscles may ultimately cause collapse of the arch and loss of stability, which results in forming the 'rocker bottom' or Charcot's foot, where a loss of sensation and weakened muscles cause bones in the foot to fracture or break when stressed. As you may not feel the damage, subsequently you may not heal properly and this can result in the shape of the foot becoming distorted. Your podiatrist will know more about treatments for this. [12]

5. Autonomic neuropathy

The final type of nerve problem is an "autonomic neuropathy." In this type of neuropathy, the nerves that control sweating are damaged. Dry skin occurs as a result of damage to these nerves. Sweating is important for heat reduction but it is also important for skin moisture balance. Without sweat, the skin dries out and cracks. This can be dangerous because germs can enter through the cracks and cause infection. Dry and cracked skin should be treated with prescription moisturizing creams and regular professional foot care. Autonomic neuropathy is a form of polyneuropathy which affects the non-voluntary, non-sensory nervous system (i.e., the autonomic nervous system) affecting mostly the internal organs such as the bladder muscles, the cardiovascular system, the digestive tract, and the genital organs. These nerves are not under a person's conscious control and function automatically. Autonomic nerve fibers form large collections in the thorax, abdomen and pelvis outside spinal cord, however they have connections with the spinal cord and ultimately the brain. Most commonly autonomic neuropathy is seen in persons with long-standing diabetes mellitus type 1 and 2. In most but not all cases, autonomic neuropathy occurs alongside other forms of neuropathy, such as sensory neuropathy.

Autonomic neuropathy is one cause of malfunction of the autonomic nervous system, but not the only one; some conditions affecting the brain or spinal cord can also cause autonomic dysfunction, such as multiple system atrophy, and therefore cause similar symptoms to autonomic neuropathy.

The signs and symptoms of autonomic neuropathy include the following:

• Urinary bladder conditions: bladder incontinence or urine retention

• Gastrointestinal tract: dysphagia, abdominal pain, nausea, vomiting, malabsorption, fecal incontinence, gastroparesis, diarrhea, constipation

• Cardiovascular system: disturbances of heart rate (tachycardia, bradycardia), orthostatic hypotension, inadequate increase of heart rate on exertion

• Other areas: hypoglycemia unawareness, genital impotence, sweat disturbances. [9]

6. Diabetic neuropathy

Most diabetics experience some type of neuropathy, a leading predisposing factor to development of ulcers. More than 60% of diabetic foot ulcers are the result of underlying neuropathy. [11,13] Diabetics have altered peripheral sensation of the foot, with loss of the protective sensation that renders the individual unaware of the beginning of an ulcer or the actual ulceration process. Diabetic neuropathy also alters the microcirculation of the foot, resulting in a reduced distribution of blood to the areas of need. Nerve damage in diabetic neuropathy occurs when blood sugar is poorly controlled for prolonged periods of time. Involvement of these nerves results in loss of the normal protective sensation that we rely upon to avoid injury. Loss of the normal pain threshold may result in prolonged and repetitive trauma to the foot. Overcompensation by other muscles can lead to other foot deformities including 'hammer' or 'claw' toes. These abnormalities lead to pressure points that are then at great risk for ulceration. Even the dry, brittle skin caused by diminished sweating is due to neuropathy affecting specialized nerves within the skin. This makes the skin prone to cracking and fissuring, thus allowing entry of bacteria even in the absence of a large sore. Subsequent infection and abscess formation may damage far more tissue than is apparent from the overlying ulcer.

The development of neuropathy in affected patients has been shown in animal and *in vitro* models to be a result of hyperglycemia-induced metabolic abnormalities. One of the more commonly described mechanisms of action is the polyol pathway. In the development of neuropathy, the hyperglycemic state leads to an increase in action of the enzymes aldose reductase and sorbitol dehydrogenase. This results in the conversion of intracellular glucose to sorbitol and fructose. The accumulation of these sugar products results in a decrease in the synthesis of nerve cell myoinositol, required for normal neuron conduction. Additionally, the chemical conversion of glucose results in a depletion of nicotinamide adenine dinucleotide phosphate stores, which are necessary for the detoxification of reactive oxygen species and for the synthesis of the vasodilator nitric oxide. There is a resultant increase in oxidative stress on the nerve cell and an increase in vasoconstriction leading to ischemia, which will promote nerve cell injury and death. Hyperglycemia and oxidative stress also contribute to the abnormal glycation of nerve cell proteins and the inappropriate activation of protein kinase C, resulting in further nerve dysfunction and ischemia.

Neuropathy in diabetic patients is manifested in the motor, autonomic, and sensory components of the nervous system. [14] Damage to the innervations of the intrinsic foot muscles leads to an imbalance between flexion and extension of the affected foot. This produces anatomic foot deformities that create abnormal bony prominences and pressure points, which gradually cause skin breakdown and ulceration.

As trauma occurs at the affected site, patients are often unable to detect the insult to their lower extremities. As a result, many wounds go unnoticed and progressively worsen as the affected area is continuously subjected to repetitive pressure and shear forces from ambulation and weight bearing. [15-20]

7. Vascular disease

Peripheral arterial disease is a contributing factor to the development of foot ulcers in up to 50% of cases. [21] It commonly affects the tibial and peroneal arteries of the calf. Endothelial cell dysfunction and smooth cell abnormalities develop in peripheral arteries as a consequence of the persistent hyperglycemic state. [22] There is a resultant decrease in endothelium-derived vasodilators leading to constriction. Further, the hyperglycemia in diabetes is associated with an increase in thromboxane A2, a vasoconstrictor and platelet aggregation agonist, which leads to an increased risk for plasma hypercoagulability. [23] There is also the potential for alterations in the vascular extracellular matrix leading to stenosis of the arterial lumen. [23] Moreover, smoking, hypertension, and hyperlipidemia are other factors that are common in diabetic patients and contribute to the development of peripheral arterial disease. [14] Cumulatively, this leads to occlusive arterial disease that results in ischemia in the lower extremity and an increased risk of ulceration in diabetic patients.

8. The extracellular matrix, fibroblast and keratinocyte

The extracellular matrix (ECM) is the non-cellular component present within all tissues and organs, and not only does provides essential physical scaffolding for the cellular constituents but also initiates crucial biochemical and biomechanical cues that are required for tissue morphogenesis, differentiation and homeostasis. The importance of the ECM is vividly illustrated by the wide range of syndromes, which can be anything from minor to severe, that arise from genetic abnormalities in ECM proteins. Although, fundamentally, the ECM is composed of water, proteins and polysaccharides, each tissue has an ECM with a unique composition and topology that is generated during tissue development through a dynamic and reciprocal, biochemical and biophysical dialogue between the various cellular components (e.g. epithelial, fibroblast, adipocyte, endothelial elements) and the evolving cellular and protein microenvironment. Indeed, the physical, topological, and biochemical composition of the ECM is not only tissue-specific, but is also markedly heterogeneous. Cell adhesion to the ECM is mediated by ECM receptors, such as integrins, discoidin domain receptors and syndecans. Adhesion mediates cytoskeletal coupling to the ECM and is involved in cell migration through the ECM. Moreover, the ECM is a highly dynamic structure that is constantly being remodeled, either enzymatically or non-enzymatically, and its molecular components are subjected to a myriad of post-translational modifications. Through these physical and biochemical characteristics the ECM generates the biochemical and mechanical properties of each organ, such as its tensile and compressive strength and elasticity, and also mediates protection by a buffering action that maintains extracellular homeostasis and water retention. In addition, the ECM directs essential morphological organization and physiological function by binding growth factors (GFs) and interacting with cell-surface receptors to elicit signal transduction and regulate gene transcription.

A fibroblast is a type of cell that synthesizes the extracellular matrix and collagen, the structural framework (stroma) for animal tissues, and plays a critical role in wound healing. Fibroblasts are the most common cells of connective tissue in animals. Inactive fibroblasts, which are also called fibrocytes, are smaller and spindle shaped. Although disjointed and scattered when they have to cover a large space, fibroblasts when crowded often locally align in parallel clusters.

Fibroblasts make collagens, glycosaminoglycans, reticular and elastic fibers, glycoproteins found in the extracellular matrix and cytokine TSLP. Growing individuals' fibroblasts are dividing and synthesizing ground substance. Tissue damage stimulates fibrocytes and induces the mitosis of fibroblasts. Unlike the epithelial cells lining the body structures, fibroblasts do not form flat monolayers and are not restricted by a polarizing attachment to a basal lamina on one side, although they may contribute to basal lamina components in some situations Fibroblasts can also migrate slowly over substratum as individual cells, again in contrast to epithelial cells. While epithelial cells form the lining of body structures, it is fibroblasts and related connective tissues which sculpt the "bulk" of an organism.

Keratinocyte is the predominant cell type in the epidermis, the outermost layer of the skin, constituting 95% of the cells found there. Those keratinocytes found in the basal layer (Stratum germinativum) of the skin are sometimes referred to as "basal cells" or "basal keratinocytes.

Wounds to the skin will be repaired in part by the migration of keratinocytes to fill in the gap created by the wound. The first set of keratinocytes to participate in that repair come from the bulge region of the hair follicle and will only survive transiently. Within the healed epidermis they will be replaced by keratinocytes originating from the epidermis. At the opposite, epidermal keratinocytes, can contribute to *de novo* hair follicle formation during the healing of large wounds. Keratinocytes migrate with a rolling motion during the process of wound healing.

9. Extracellular matrix, fibroblast and keratinocyte in diabetic foot ulcer

Diabetic nephropathy (DN) is a serious complication in diabetes and is characterized by excessive deposition of extracellular matrix proteins in the mesangium and basement membrane. Major typical morphological changes are the result of changes in the extracellular matrix (ECM). One important ECM component, the proteoglycans (PGs), shows a more complex pattern of changes in DN. PGs in basement membranes are decreased. The amounts and structures of heparan sulfate chains are changed, and such changes affect levels of growth factors regulating cell proliferation and ECM synthesis, with cell attachment affecting endothelial cells. Enzymes modulating heparan sulfate structures, such as heparanase and sulfatases, are implicated in DN. Other enzyme classes also modulate ECM proteins and PGs, such as matrix metalloproteinases and serine proteases, such as plasminogen activator, as well as their corresponding inhibitors. The levels of these enzymes and inhibitors are changed in plasma and in the kidneys in DN. Several growth factors, signaling pathways, and hyperglycemia per se affect ECM synthesis and turnover in DN. Therefore, ECM components are being evaluated to be used as markers for DN. [24-27]

10. Matrix metalloproteinases

Matrix metalloproteinases (MMPs) are a family of nine or more highly homologous $Zn(++)$-endopeptidases that collectively cleave most if not all of the constituents of the extracellular matrix.

In diabetic foot ulcers there is an excess of MMPs and a decrease of the tissue inhibitors of MMPs (TIMPs). This imbalance is probably one cause of impaired healing. However, little is known about changes in MMPs during wound healing. A high level of MMP-1 seems essential to wound healing, while an excess of MMP-8 and -9 is deleterious, and could be a target for new topical treatments. The MMP-1/TIMP-1 ratio is a predictor of wound healing in diabetic foot ulcers. [28]

11. Risk factors in diabetic foot

Early recognition and management of risk factors is important for reducing morbidity of foot ulceration. These risk factors, as investigated by several teams, [29-33] include age, sex (being male), diabetes duration and type, insulin use, past history of diabetic foot ulcer (DFU) and amputation, lower limb bypass procedures, biomechanical factors such as glycaemia level and poor glycaemic control, dyslipidaemia, sensory and autonomic neuropathy (foot insensitivity to the 5.07 monofilament), absence of reflex and limited joint motion, muscle weakness, callus formation, Charcot deformity, hammer/claw toe deformity, abnormal Achilles tendon reflex, greater body mass (≥20kg), arterial insufficiency, vascular disease, skin dryness and fissure (caused by autonomic neuropathy), reduced skin oxygenation and foot perfusion (defined as ankle-brachial index ABI<0.9, toe systolic pressure <45 mmHg, 13mmHg orthostatic blood pressure fall and 15mmHg higher dorsal foot transcutaneous PO2), diastolic hypertension, impaired vision, as well as socio-environmental risk factors in some communities, such as smoking habits, alcohol consumptions, lack of proper diabetes educations, low income, racial distribution (African Americans, Hispanic Americans and Native Americans face a higher risk), poor personal hygiene and self-care.

Smoking, hypertension, and hyperlipidemia are considered as risk factors due to their effects on the increased occurrence of peripheral arterial occlusive disease in diabetics, which typically involves the tibial and peroneal arteries, but leaves the dorsalis pedis artery unaffected. [14]

There are controversies on some other factor, as some studies could not find a relationship between them and DFU occurrence. They include height, hallux blood pressure, and other foot deformities. [34,35] Also, although some studies could not find a statistically significant association between the length of diabetes and the risk of DFU, other studies mentioned it could be predictive. [36]

Wounds that are penetrated to bone, wounds older than 30 days, recurrent wounds, and presence of peripheral vascular disease increase the risk of wound infections. [37]

The majority (80%) of DFUs is the consequences of neuropathies due to decreasing pain sensation and perception of pressure, to causing muscle imbalance that can lead to anatomic deformities, and to impairing the microcirculation and the integrity of the skin. Therefore, risk factors in neuropathy should also be considered as risk factors in DFU. They include unbalanced age, sex (male gender), duration of diabetes, higher glycemia level, higher levels of LDL and triglycerides, higher von Willebrand factor levels and urinary albumin excretion rate, hypertension, depression and atherosclerosis (ischemia). [34,38,39]

12. Symptoms and prediction

Diabetic foot ulcers usually start with the following symptoms:

- Atrophic integument
- Any break in the skin resulted from abnormal wear and tear, injury, or infection
- Sores, ulcers, or blisters on the foot or lower leg
- Persistent pain, which can be a symptom of sprain, strain, bruise, overuse, improperly fitting shoes, or underlying infection.
- Calluses and corns that may be a sign of chronic trauma to the foot
- A claudicating or difficulty walking that can be sign of joint problems, serious infection, or improperly fitting shoes
- Discoloration in feet: black, blue, or red
- Cold feet

- Absent pulses

- Swollen foot or ankle

- Odor

- Fever or chills in association with a wound that can be a sign of a limb-threatening or life-threatening infection

- Redness, which can be a sign of infection, especially when surrounding a wound, or of abnormal rubbing of shoes or socks.

- Swelling of the feet or legs, which can be a sign of underlying inflammation or infection, improperly fitting shoes, or poor venous circulation.

- New or lasting numbness in the feet or legs, a sign of nerve damage from diabetes

- Signs of poor blood circulation, such as:

  ○ Pain in the legs that increases with walking but improves with rest (claudication)

  ○ Absence of pedal hair or pallor on elevation (coupled with other symptoms)

  ○ Hard shiny skin on the legs

  ○ Toenail fungus, athlete's foot, and ingrown toenails, which may lead to more serious bacterial infections

- Drainage of pus from a wound is usually a sign of infection. Persistent bloody drainage is also a sign of a potentially serious foot problem.

13. Classification of foot ulcers

Several schemes have been used to classify diabetic foot ulcers, but none of them has been accepted universally. Following is a list of the most used classifications: [40]

Wagner-Meggitt, the most popular method that was described by Meggitt (1976) and Wagner (1982), [41,42] has been used for decades to classify DFUs in six grades based on the wound's depths and extent of gangrene (table 2):

Grade 0	Intact skin (only foot symptoms like pain exist)
Grade 1	Superficial ulcer
Grade 2	Deep ulcer to tendon, bone or joint
Grade 3	Deep ulcer with abscess or osteomyelitis
Grade 4	Forefoot gangrene
Grade 5	Whole foot gangrene

Table 2. Wagner-Meggitt grades of diabetic foot ulcer classification.

University of Texas classification, which has been developed by Armstrong and his colleagues, is a more comprehensive scale and includes risk stratification and expresses tissue breakdown, infection and gangrene separately (table 3). [42] The University of Texas scale showed a better correlation with prognosis and risk of amputation: [14]

Grade 0	Pre-ulcerative site, or healed ulcer.
Grade 1	Ulcer through the epidermis +/- dermis, but not to tendon, capsule or bone
	1A- without infection or ischaemia
	1B- with infection but no ischaemia
	1C- with ischaemia
	1D- with ischaemia and infection
Grade 2	Ulcer to capsule or tendon
	2A- without infection or ischaemia
	2B- with infection but no ischaemia
	2C- with ischaemia
	2D- with ischaemia and infection
Grade 3	Ulcer to bone or joint
	3A- without infection or ischaemia
	3B- with infection but no ischaemia
	3C- with ischaemia
	3D- with ischaemia and infection

Table 3. University of Texas grades of diabetic foot ulcer classification

Although Texas classification describes the grade of wound in more details, it does not include measures of neuropathy or ulcer area.

S(AD) SAD system builds upon the Wagner classification to include several additional categories: size (area, depth), sepsis, arteriopathy and denervation. [43] Developed by an English group, the S(AD) SAD classification is a validated system with grades 0 to 3, [44] as shown in table 4:

Grade		Size	Sepsis	Arteriopathy	Denervation
Area	Depth				
0	Skin intact	Skin intact	None	Pedal pulses present	Pin pricks intact
1	< 1 cm2	Superficial (skin and subcutaneous tissue)	Surface	Pedal pulses reduced or one missing	Pin pricks reduced
2	1-3 cm2	Tendon, periosteum, joint capsule	Cellulitis	Absence of both pedal pulses	Pin pricks absent
3	> 3 cm2	Bone or joint space	Osteomyelitis	Gangrene	Charcot

Table 4. S(AD) SAD classification for diabetic foot ulcer

RYB Color Classification was developed for the nursing literature [45] and has obtained considerable popularity. The system relies purely on a color scheme with no additional considerations. R/Red wounds are those that exhibit pale pink to beefy red granulation tissue and are deemed to be in the inflammatory or proliferative phase. Y/Yellow wounds are marked by pale ivory, yellowish green or brown color, slough of necrotic but moist tissue, and wound exudates. B/Black wounds are marked by black, brown or tan color, and desiccated eschar. The RYB classification is an easy and widely accepted system in the nursing literature and shows the continuum from acute to chronic wounds. Conversely, it is non-specific with no consideration of depth or size, and no consideration of the contributing factor of neuropathy.

PEDIS classification was proposed by the International Working Group on the Diabetic Foot [46,47] and grades the wounds on the basis of five features: perfusions (arterial supply), extent (area), depth, infection and sensation. There are levels of 1 to 4 for each of these factors. The in-depth nature of this system is appropriate for the research community that desires this amount of detail. Every lesion is described (for example P2E1D2I1S2), according to table 5:

Grade	Perfusion (P)	Extent/size (E) (cm²)	Depth/tissue loss (D)	Infection (I)	Sensation (S)
1	no symptoms/ signs of PAD		Superficial full-thickness ulcer	no symptoms/signs	No loss of protective sensation
2	symptoms or signs of PAD, but not CLI		Ulcer penetrating below dermis to skin structures	Inflammation of skin only	Loss of protective sensation
3	CLI		All subsequent layers of foot, including bone/ joint	Extensive erythema deeper than skin	
4				Systemic inflammatory response syndrome (SIRS)	

Table 5. Grades of PEDIS classification for diabetic foot ulcer

Determination of the level of infection in PEDIS classification system is based on the Severity Classification guideline published by the Infectious Disease Society of America (IDSA), as shown in table 6:

Clinical Manifestation of Infection	Infection Severity	PEDIS Grade
Wound lacking purulence or any manifestations of inflammation.	Uninfected	1
Presence of ≥ 2 manifestations of inflammation (purulence, or erythema, pain, tenderness, warmth, or induration), but any cellulitis/erythema extends ≤ 2 cm around the ulcer, and infection is limited to the skin or superficial subcutaneous tissues; no other local complications or systemic illness.	Mild	2
Infection (as above) in a patient who is systemically well and metabolically stable, but which has ≥ 1 of the following characteristics: cellulitis extending > 2 cm, lymphangitic streaking, spread beneath the superficial fascia, deep-tissue abscess, gangrene, and involvement of muscle, tendon, joint, or bone.	Moderate	3
Infection in a patient with systemic toxicity or metabolic instability (e.g., fever, chills, tachycardia, hypotension, confusion, vomiting, leukocytosis, acidosis, severe hyperglycemia, or azotemia).	Severe	4

Table 6. Severity classification guideline according to IDSA

DEPA Scoring System, is the newest DFU classification system, in which D stands for depth of the ulcer, E for extent of bacterial colonization, P for phase of ulcer, and A for associated etiology (table 7). [48] Ascending scores, from 1 to 3, are assigned for increasing levels of intensity in each category (see the table below). For instance, an ulcer involving soft tissue receives a 2. Contamination of this ulcer receives a 1. The ulcer is in the inflammatory phase, generating a 2 score, and has an underlying bony deformity, generating another 2 score. Accordingly, this ulcer has a total score of 7. Ulcers with a total score of 6 or less are considered "low grade" ulcers. Recommended treatment measures include oral antibiotics (if infected), blood sugar control (type not specified) and debridement. Those with a total score of 7 to 9 are deemed "moderate grade" wounds that one would treat with parenteral antibiotics, insulin, debridement, healing promoting agents and pressure relieving methods. The "high grade" lesions, those with a total score between 10 and 12, require a conservative trial including parenteral antibiotics, insulin, debridement, healing promoting agents and vascular reconstruction. The authors of the DEPA classification system offered acute ischemia patients a below-knee amputation; however, other practitioners may offer revascularization or other interventions. The scores of 11 to 12 are prognostic for amputation and if these are heel ulcers, they were even more likely to lead to amputation. Scores of 10 or greater predict difficulty with healing, while scores of 6 or less indicate probable healing.

DEPA Score	Score		
	1	2	3
Depth of the ulcer	Skin	Soft tissue	Bone
Extent of bacterial colonization	Contamination	Infection	Necrotizing infection[a]
Phase of ulcer	Granulating[b]	Inflammatory[c]	Nonhealing[d]
Associated etiology	Neuropathy	Bone deformity	Ischemia[e]

[a] Infected ulcer with surrounding cellulitis or fasciitis.

[b] Evidence of granulation tissue formation.

[c] Hyperemic ulcer with no granulation tissue <2 weeks' duration.

[d] Nongranulating ulcer >2 weeks' duration.

[e] Clinical signs and symptoms of chronic lower-limb ischemia.

Table 7. Scores and definitions of DEPA scoring system

14. Vascular impaired in foot ulcers

Vascular impairment is one of the most important causes of DFU, and in addition to hyperglycemia, is the main impediment in healing the ulcers. Smoking cessation, diet improvement and controlling total and LDL cholesterol, antiplatelet drug treatment, and maintaining an optimum blood pressure will help reducing the impact of vascular impairment on ulcer healing. Vascular impairment in foot ulcers has been discussed in more details in 7.

15. Angiogenesis in foot ulcer

When a tissue is injured, blood from the broken capillaries streams into the wound. This blood carries platelets and fibrinogen. Fibrinogen is activated in response to the exposed epithelium to form a fibrin mesh that traps platelets. Platelets also adhere to the ruptured blood vessels, preventing further blood loss. Moreover, platelets come into contact with damaged ECM components; they release clotting factors, leading to the formation of a blood clot within the wound site. The activated platelets in the wound release chemical stimuli such as platelet-derived growth factor (PDGF), transforming growth factor-β (TGF-β), and vascular endothelial growth factor (VEGF). [49,50] Fibroblasts stimulated by these chemoattractants produce collagen, which is a major component of the ECM, a scaffold onto which the endothelial cells can migrate to create and extend the vascular network. Fibroblasts also secrete PDGF and TGF-β, as well as VEGF. This cocktail of growth factors stimulates the endothelial cells of vessels in the nearby healthy tissue to release proteases such as MMPs. [51] MMPs digest the basement membrane, allowing endothelial cells to escape the confines of their parent vessels. [52] VEGF, EGF, bFGF, and TGF-β stimulate the systematic rearrangement of endothelial cells from blood vessels. The cells proliferate, elongate, and align to form a capillary sprout, extending away from the original vessel. [49] This is the beginning of the angiogenesis process. Then, polarized endothelial cells are positioned with a luminal and an abluminal surface forming tubular structures, which act as a multipurpose barrier between the flowing blood and the extravascular tissue. Periendothelial cells, such as pericytes, fibroblasts, and smooth muscle cells, reinforce these tubular endothelial networks. This process is oxygen dependent. Oxygen is required for collagen deposition. Hypoxia causes the hypoxia-inducible factor (HIF) to up-regulate the production of VEGF.

Sprout extension is facilitated by endothelial cell proliferation and further migration toward the chemical attractant.

Vasculogenesis, the formation of blood vessels from the differentiation of progenitor cells, also plays a part in the formation of new blood vessels during this stage of wound healing. [53] Progenitor cells differentiate into early endothelial progenitor cells in the bone marrow and further differentiate into late endothelial progenitor cells in the vasculature system before arriving at the site of vessel formation. [52]

The joining of two capillary sprouts within a healing wound forms a loop through which blood can flow and new sprouts develop from this vessel thus propagating angiogenesis. [54] This capillary extension allows oxygen and other critical nutrients to be transported further into the injured region. This, in turn, allows the macrophage and fibroblast fronts to migrate further into the wound, and thus the healing unit progresses into the injured tissue. [54] When the unit has completely swept through the wound site, blood vessels are networked over the entire space and oxygen levels are returned to normal. Oxygen binds to HIF and leads to a decreased synthesis of VEGF. This ends the angiogenesis process. [49]

Usually diabetes causes excessive and deficient angiogenesis (table 8). Therapeutic factors that can regulate angiogenesis in the diabetic foot conditions are considered as successful treatments for DFU.

16. Diagnostic tests and prediction

A task force of the Foot Care Interest Group of the American Diabetes Association (ADA) released a report in 2008 that specifies recommended components of foot examinations for patients with diabetes (table 9). [55]

Defective angiogenesis		Excessive angiogenesis	
Phenotype	Causes	Phenotype	Causes
Reduced angiogenesis and collateral formation	Reduced VEGF, FGF, EPC circulation, cytokines, ECM/BM degradation; increased AGEs and MMP	Retinal capillary occlusion	Elevated intraocular pressure
Vascular occlusion, inflammation	Increased free fatty acids, polyol pathway, cytokines, ICAM, VCAM	Increased vascular permeability	Increased VEGF
Reduced wound healing; transplant failure	Reduced VEGF and growth factors; sorbitol-inositol imbalance; increased ACE, Ang-II and tissue factor mRNA	Capillary sprouting	Increased VEGF, FGF, PDGF; cytokines (TGF-β); integrins
Embryonic vasculopathy (anomalous vasculogenesis and angiogenesis)	Reduced VEGF, IL-1, TGF-β	Vascular remodeling	Increased laminin, fibronectin, collagen IV, ECM components, lipidosis

Table 8. Comparison of aberrant angiogenesis under diabetes.

Risk Category	Definition	Treatment Recommendation	Suggested Follow-up
0	No LOPS, no PAD, no deformity	Consider patient education on foot care, including information on appropriate footwear.	Annually (by generalist and/or specialist)
1	LOPS±deformity	Consider prescriptive or accommodative footwear. Consider prophylactic surgery if deformity is not able to be safely accommodated in shoes. Continue patient education.	Every 3-6 months (by generalist or specialist)
2	PAD±LOPS	Consider the use of accommodative footwear. Consider a vascular consultation for combined follow-up.	Every 2-3 months (by specialist)
3	History of ulcer or amputation	Consider patient education on foot care. Consider vascular consultation for combined follow-up if PAD present.	Every 1-2 months (by specialist)

LOPS, loss of protective sensation; PAD, peripheral arterial disease. Adapted from [55]

Table 9. Risk classification system of the Task Force of the Foot Care Interest Group of the ADA

Foot deformity is an important diagnostic sign for future foot ulcer. In addition to Charcot arthropathy, hyperextension of the metatarsal-phalangeal joint with interphalangeal or distal phalangeal joint flexion leads to hammer toe and claw toe deformities, respectively. The deformities may lead to ulceration by continuous improper contact with the footwear.

In examining for vascular abnormalities of the foot, the dorsalis pedis and posterior tibial pulses should be palpated and characterized as present or absent. Claudication, loss of hair, and the presence of pale, thin, shiny, or cool skin are physical findings suggestive of potential ischemia. [56] If vascular disease is a concern, measuring the ankle brachial index (ABI) can be used in the outpatient setting for determining the extent of vascular disease and need for referral to a vascular specialist. The ABI is obtained by measuring the systolic blood pressures in the ankles (dorsalis pedis and posterior tibial arteries) and arms (brachial artery) using a handheld Doppler and then calculating a ratio. However, in patients with calcified, poorly compressible vessels or aortoiliac stenosis, the results of the ABI can be complicated. [57]

The loss of pressure sensation in the foot has to be identified using a 10-guage monofilament as a significant predictive factor for the likelihood of ulceration. [57]

High vibration perception thresholds (VPTs) using a biothesiometer or a tuning fork, high plantar pressure and 10-gauge monofilaments are used as reliable methods to identify those at risk of future ulceration. [36]

17. Foot amputation

Despite all efforts to treat ischemic and neuropathic ulcers, sometimes the lower-extremity is non-viable and amputation is inevitable. Non-traumatic amputations are high in poorer countries and in uneducated people in wealthy countries. Amputees suffer from direct surgical morbidity and mortality, inadequate and delayed rehabilitation. Also, amputees attract great amount of care from a multidisciplinary team and put additional pressure on countries' health systems and disability insurances.

The indications for amputation in patients with diabetes are often multiple, mostly a non-healing ulcer, or frequent gangrene and infection occurring simultaneously. [58] Whether primary minor amputation is beneficial in comparison with primary major amputation (below knee) is still controversial. Digital toe amputation eventually leads to limb loss, while a major amputation lowers the risk of re-amputation. [59] Re-amputation widely rates from 21% to 60%, and is greatest in the first 6 to 12 months after the first amputation. [60,61] Once hallux has gone under amputation, changes in mechanical force and pressure on the foot may increase the likelihood of developing further lesions, most probably within 6 months. [62] Studies by Byrne et al. 1992 and Yeager et al. 1998 showed that revascularization may not prevent re-amputation as patients undergoing revascularization procedures are likely to have severe ischaemic disease. [63,64]

18. Treatments

Any diabetic patient with a skin break below the knee that has not healed with appropriate care in 2 weeks should be referred urgently to a suitable specialist for an assessment. Assessment of the cause of an ulcer helps clinicians in determining the most appropriate treatment. The assessment includes testing for sensation, palpating for foot pulses, measuring the ankle-brachial pressure index (ABPI) and toe pressures, and often undertaking color-flow duplex ultrasonography. Patients with lower-limb tissue loss from ischemia should be assessed by a vascular surgeon. Magnetic resonance angiography (MRA) or conventional intra-arterial digital subtraction angiography could be needed to help plan the reconstruction. [65-68]

DFU can be successfully treated by a multidisciplinary team consists of diabetologist, shoemaker, orthopedist, psychologist, vascular and general surgeons, podologists, radiologists, educators, nurses and rehabilitation team. [35]

Surgeons (general, vascular, orthopaedic, plastic, podiatric) generally become involved in treating severe tissue infection, especially when gangrene or underlying osteomyelitis remain despite antibiotic treatment. [69] The main purpose of surgery is to remove infected and necrotic soft and bony tissue back to a healthy base that will support granulation tissue and allow healing by secondary intention.

Many diabetic patients with underlying ischemia will need revascularization to provide an adequate arterial blood supply in order to achieve a better healing and resolve underlying infection. Up to a 90% 10-year limb-salvage rate has been demonstrated with surgical bypass procedures of the lower extremity. [70] A standard treatment for ischemic ulceration is still femorodistal bypass with an autogenous tissue (usually saphenous vein), although this treatment is not readily available for all patients. However, it seems reasonable to attempt healing of ischemic and neuroischemic ulcers with drugs before considering revascularization.

Conventional treatments for diabetic peripheral neuropathy include tricyclic compounds, serotonin-norepinephrine reuptake inhibitors (e.g. duloxtine), anticonvulsants (e.g. pregabalin), opiates, membrane stabilizers, the antioxidant alpha lipoic acid and others. [33]

The selection of wound dressings is also an important component of diabetic wound care management. Advanced wound dressing products can help alter the wound environment to optimize healing conditions. Characteristics of a successful wound dressing will be discussed later.

If not managed properly, diabetic foot ulcers are at high risk for infection. Open wounds can be contaminated or infected with microorganisms and even virulent pathogens. The generally accepted clinical definition of infection is the presence of purulent secretions or at least two signs or symptoms of inflammation (erythema, warmth, tenderness, pain, and induration). While ischemia or neuropathy signs such as friable tissue, wound undermining, and foul odor imply infection. [71] Most diabetic foot infections do not produce systemic signs, such as fever or leukocytosis, but when they are present, they typically suggest that any accompanying infection is severe.

To assess the infection, clinicians should obtain material for a wound culture. Tissue specimens are strongly preferred to wound swabs, because they provide more sensitive and specific results. Tissue can be obtained by scraping of the base of the ulcer with a scalpel or dermal curette (curettage) or by wound biopsy. Aseptically obtained aspirates of pus (purulent secretions) or tissue fluid can also provide good specimens for culture. The specimen should be processed for both aerobic and anaerobic cultures and a gram-stained smear, if possible. Blood obtained for a complete blood count (and leucocyte differential), basic serum chemistry panels, and inflammatory markers (erythrocyte sedimentation rate [ESR] or C-reactive protein) can help define the severity of the infection. [72]

Usually, plain radiographs of the foot will help to identify foreign bodies, gas in the tissues, or evidence of osteomyelitis. More sophisticated imaging tests (the best of which being MRI) might be needed to better define the presence or absence of bone or deep soft-tissue infection.

Infection of bone underlying a foot ulcer is an especially difficult diagnostic and therapeutic problem. Osteomyelitis is probably present if the bone is visible or palpable by probing. Bone infection must usually be present for at least 2 weeks before it can be regarded as the cause of abnormalities seen on plain radiographs. Most nuclear medicine tests (e.g., technetium bone scans or labeled leucocyte scans) are more sensitive than plain radiography, but are relatively non-specific and less accurate than MRI. The gold standard test for osteomyelitis is a bone biopsy sample processed for culture and histology. [73]

All available data are required to decide whether infections are safe to treat on an outpatient basis, or whether hospital care is needed for medical, diagnostic, surgical, or psychosocial reasons. [30]

Antibiotics are selected largely based on the probable causative organisms, taking into account any known local antibiotic resistance patterns. Patients with severe infections need parenteral treatment, at least initially; oral therapy is often adequate for those with mild or moderate infections. [74]

Topical antimicrobials are often effective for mildly infected ulcers, however, some topical antiseptics can impair wound healing, but dressings containing silver or iodine seem to be safe, and possibly useful (see later). [75]

The aim of antimicrobial therapy is to cure the infection, not to heal the wound; extended treatment increases the risk of drug-related toxic effects and development of antibiotic resistance. Antibiotic treatment without off-loading a plantar wound (i.e., the relieving of a mechanical load) is unlikely to result in ulcer healing (see later).

Bone infection is best treated by surgical resection of all infected and necrotic bone, but retrospective studies suggest that long-term treatment (at least for 4–6 weeks) with drugs that penetrate well into bone (e.g., fluoroquinolones) can often produce a remission of infection. [73]

19. Treatment-based classification system for the diabetic foot

Recently developed treatments for diabetic foot ulcers include the use of bone marrow-derived stem cells, [76] use of human or bioengineered skin equivalents, [77,78] growth-factor therapy (such as using PDGF or G-CSF) [79,80] and negative pressure wound therapy (NPWT) [81]. Hyperbaric oxygen treatment (HBOT) seems to reduce the risk of major amputation, but not the time to ulcer healing or the rate of minor amputation. [82,83] Routine debridement of devitalized tissue at follow-up visits is widely recommended. [84] Maggot (larval) biotherapy seems to be effective for debridement [85] and acceleration of healing, [86,87] and perhaps also in reducing antibiotic use and risk of amputation. [88] A recently developed natural-based medicine, ANGIPARS™, has shown excellent effects on wound closure and shortening the wound healing period in both diabetic foot ulcers [89-93] and pressure ulcers, [94,95] via strong angiogenesis, anti-oxidant, [96] anti-coagulant and properties.

Negative Pressure Wound Therapy (NPWT) is a sealed wound-care system and is particularly indicated for a large chronic persistent wounds and acute complicated wounds. The system consists of an electronically controlled pump and a foam dressing that drains the wound. [97] An adjustable negative pressure is applied via an airtight adhesive film that covers the wound. NPWT drains wound exudates and is thought to promote blood circulation and healing. [98] NPWT benefits include increased local blood flow, [99] rapid wound granulation, increased number of active fibroblasts and macrophages, [99] epithelial isolation, migration and contraction, [94,95] reduction of dressing changes, [100] reduced infection risk, [101] reduced treatment costs, [59] control of exudates that contain harmful fluid and by-products of tissue damage, [99,102] concurrent rehabilitation, [103] and better patient tolerance. [104] However, it is impossible to conclude from the studies that NPWT performs absolutely or relatively better than the control treatments in terms of wound healing. [105] Only one study showed a statistically significant difference in wound healing in the test group compared to the control. Although a few studies showed some NPWT effect in shortening the wound closure time, its total efficacy cannot be fully concluded because the studies were not properly designed in terms of methods of measurement, blinding and follow-ups. [106] There was high potential for bias and diagnostic heterogeneity in the studies. To approve if NPWT has a positive effect on wound healing, further research clinical trials of good methodological quality are required. Moreover, the FDA recently issued a report on six deaths and 77 other complications that were reported within a two-year period in connection with NPWT. All the deaths were caused by acute hemorrhages, and known contraindications for NPWT (e.g. a large blood vessel exposed) had clearly been overlooked. Many of the deaths occurred in outpatient care or care homes, which highlights the need to monitor therapy. [59,107]

Hyperbaric Oxygen Treatment (HBOT), which is used for Wagner Grade 3 diabetic wounds that have failed to resolve after a 30-day course of standard treatment, is the delivery of pure oxygen to patients at higher than normal atmospheric pressures to compensate shortage of blood oxygen due to vascular impairment. [83] The usual pressure for treating DFU is 1.4 to 3 atmospheres absolute pressure (ATA) - with an optimum of 2 ATA - for a compression time of 60 to 120 minutes - with an optimum of 90 minutes - during a course of multiple treatments.

[97,108,109] This high pressure results in an increase in the concentration of oxygen in the blood and an increase in the diffusion capacity to the tissues, which, in turn, stimulates neovascularization and fibroblast replication and increases phagocytosis and leukocyte-mediated killing of bacterial pathogens in the wound. [109] A long benefits list of increasing the tissue oxygen is made through several studies [50]: modulation of the production of nitric oxide, promotion of cellular proliferation, stimulation of capillary budding, alteration of ischemic effect, modification of the effect of growth factors and cytokines, acceleration of collagen deposition, reduction of edema, modulation of the immune system response, accelerated microbial oxidative killing, and enhancement of oxygen radical scavengers, thereby reducing ischemia reperfusion injury.

There is enough good evidence that HBOT decreases risk of amputation in patients with complicated or infected DFU. [110,111] Many studies have shown that HBOT results in partial or complete wound healing. Some studies also showed that HBOT in combination with surgery and antibiotics can be used to treat refractory osteomyelitis. HBOT is reasonably safe when administered by experienced practitioners after careful patient screening and selection. [112]

Wound dressing, widely used to cure the infected wounds, is the most important component of a successful wound care. There are a number of available dressing types to consider. Although there is a shortage of published trials to support the use of one type of dressing compared to another, [113] the characteristics of specific dressing types can prove beneficial depending on the characteristics of the individual wound. An ideal dressing should contribute to a moist wound environment, absorb excessive exudates, and not increase the risk for infections. [114] Dressing changes and wound inspection should occur on a daily basis. [113] Saline-soaked gauze dressings, for example, are inexpensive, well tolerated, and contribute to an atraumatic, moist wound environment. Foam and alginate dressings are highly absorbent and can aid in decreasing the risk for maceration in wounds with heavy exudates.

The process of autolysis is important in wound care. If an occlusive dressing is provided as a barrier to the outside environment, the body's own phagocytic processes will provide debridement of wounds. These products range from occlusive films such as Tegaderm, which are permeable to air and water vapor, but impermeable to fluid and microorganisms to hydrocolloids such as DuoDerm, which are also occlusive but provide absorption of exudates in addition to maintaining a moist environment for autolysis. For heavily exudative wounds, there are a range of absorptive products, including various hydrophilic foam dressings, hydrogels, hydrofibers, and alginates, which can absorb up to 20 times their weight. [115]

Silver dressings have been used for decades with little significant toxicity to cure infected wounds. Silver has a very broad spectrum of microbial coverage, including yeast, fungi, mold, and even antibiotic-resistant organisms, when used at appropriate concentrations. Silver ion binds to negatively charged particles such as proteins, DNA, RNA and chloride ions. [116,117] Introduced in 1968, silver sulfadiazine is known to release active silver ion gradually for a longer time. [118] Nanocrystalline silver dressing developed since 1990s to fix the shortcomings of this type of dressing. It contains two layers of high-density polyethylene net sandwiching a layer of rayon/polyester gauze. The outer layer is coated with a nanocrystalline (<20 nm), uncharged form of silver, and the inner layer helps maintain a moist environment for wound healing. [116] This sandwich provides a sustained release of silver into the wound due to the low affinity of Ag0 to the negatively-charged particles in the wound. Other advantage of nanocrystalline silver dressing is less frequency of dressing changes compared the standard silver dressings, which must be changed up to 12 times a day. This brings less disruption to the wound healing bed.

Growth factors play the most important role in orchestrating the cells in wound bed along the process of wound healing. When a wound occurs, platelets and fibroblasts recruited to the wound bed, start secreting growth factors, such as PDGF, VEGF, EGF, G-CSF (GM-CSF), and TGF-β. G-CSF or GM-CSF has been found to enhance the activity of neutrophils, macrophages, keratinocytes, and fibroblasts, and increase VEGF production in diabetic patients. [119,120] A meta-analysis study revealed that, although the use of G-CSF did not significantly accelerate the resolution of infection in diabetic wounds, there was a decreased likelihood of amputation and the need for other surgical therapies in treated wounds. [121]

In a study by Steed et al., patients who were treated with recombinant human platelet-derived growth factor (rhPDGF) showed statistically significant higher percentage of wound healing (48% vs. 25% in control group), as well as greater reduction in wound size. Now, known as becaplermin or Regranex, rhPDGF is used in treatment regimens for DFU. [122,123]

Stem cell therapy has emerged as a promising treatment modality aiming to address the underlying pathophysiology of DFU. Stem cells secrete chemokines and growth factors (especially EGF, VEGF and fibronectin), which promote angiogenesis and ECM remodeling to mobilize wound healing. Stem cells that have been studied for wound healing can be classified in two groups of allogenic and autologous, based on where their origins are. Placental or amnion-derived mesenchymal stem cells and embryonic stem cells are categorized as allogenic stem cells. On the other hand, bone marrow-derived endothelial progenitor cells, bone marrow-derived mesenchymal stem cells, hematopoietic stem cells, and mesenchymal stem cells derived from adipose tissue are the autologous stem cells. [124] Placenta-derived MSCs are shown to be more effective in chronic wound healing. [125,126] Also, isolated ESC-derived EPCs were shown to improve re-epithelialization when injected subcutaneously into or applied topically on to the wound. [127] In another study, bone marrow-derived stem cells were applied on to chronic wounds that were not healed for more than a year. The treated wounds showed signs of closures within 2-4 weeks post-treatment, where there was a direct correlation between the number of cells applied and the percent decrease in wound size. [128] Another study also showed 81% limb salvage when bone marrow-derived stem cells were injected to the wounds that were otherwise candidates for amputations. [129] Hematopoietic stems cells (HSCs), harvested from either bone marrow or peripheral blood, are shown to enhance wounds healing in both the inflammatory and proliferative phases of DFU. [130] Despite promising results, the majority of these studies are conducted in animals and the few human studies are not providing enough documents to include the stem cell therapies in fixed treatments protocols of foot ulcers. More studies are required to demonstrate the safety, efficacy and improved healing rates. The main obstacle stem cell therapy strategies are facing is a proper system of delivering cells to the precise location within the wound. [124] One other major reason for limited adoption of stem cells or their products is the cost of obtaining and preparing the cells. [74]

Bioengineered skin and skin grafts have also been investigated for wound healing. Tissue-engineered skin substitutes are usually categorized in allogenic cell-containing and autologous cell-containing matrices (both carry living keratinocytes or fibroblasts), as well as acellular matrices. They all release growth factors to stimulate wound healing. [131,132] Some degrees of healing have been demonstrated through some studies, [133-138] however, because the results were susceptible to bias due to the poor methodology, more studies are required to confirm those results. [139]

ANGIPARS™, an herbal-origin drug, has shown promising results during phase II and III, and post-marketing phase IV studies. [90-93,140] The main ingredient of this medicine is an herb, called *Melilotus officinalis* (yellow sweet clover). Melilotus extracts are shown to have anti-inflammation, anti-spasmodic, aromatic, carminative, diuretic, emollient, mildly expectorant, mildly sedative and vulnerary effects. Therefore, ANGIPARS™ was expected and proved to possess angiogenesis, anti-oxidative and anti-inflammatory properties, and to be able to improve the local blood circulation and provide trace elements effective in the wound healing. Excessive studies had shown that it was effective in treating DFU and decubitus ulcer, and in preventing from amputation. In those studies, an obvious wound healing was observed after a 4-week therapy period. The Producer suggests the following indications and clinical uses: [141]

- Adult patients with diabetes type 1 and 2 suffering from single and multiple foot ulcer(s) in Wagner's grade 1 and 2, and infection-controlled grade 3.

- Patients with foot ulcers that are caused due to peripheral neuropathy or other neuropathies, foot deformities, traumas, using unsuitable shoes, history of foot ulcer or amputation, joint movement limitation, uncontrolled hyperglycemia, prolonged diabetes, etc.

A widely-collective document registration on case reports is required to confirm ANGI-PARS™ as a potent drug in DFU treatment. [74]

20. Foot care and management of foot ulcer

One of the easiest, least expensive and most effective ways for preventing foot complications could be careful inspection of the diabetic foot on a regular basis. [14]

Initial management consists of cleansing of the wound, debriding of any necrotic or gangrenous material, and the probing (preferably with a blunt sterile metal instrument) for foreign bodies or exposed bone.

There is no doubt that one of the most important parts of DFU treatments or prevention plans should be off-loading, meaning pressure relief on ulcer. High plantar pressure is usually caused by bony deformity or displacement of soft tissues, and may lead to ulceration and failure to heal. Ulcers can also be caused by contact between the dorsal surface of deformed toes and footwear that does not provide adequate toe room.

A successful off-loading through a total contact cast can decrease the pressure from 1000 kPa to less than 100 kPa. [142] Total casts should be properly made and changed at least weekly. It has been shown that patients bearing ulcer are not usually complaint with a removable off-loading device. [143] Various ambulatory braces, splints, modified shoes, and sandals can off-load the plantar surface or immobilize the foot and ankle or both. A modified half-shoe can help off-load pressure from half of the foot. Felted-foam, soft polymeric insoles and orthoses with load-isolation regions are also used to smoothen the inner layers of shoes. [144] For interdigital lesions, the close or overlapping toes must be separated. Ulcers on the plantar aspect of the heel take longer to heal than those on the forefoot in total contact casts and could benefit from special shoes without a rear-foot platform.

DFU patients are encouraged to reduce their activity levels temporarily. Patients are typically less active in total contact casts than in healing shoes, presumably because of the bulk and weight of the irremovable device. Increased activity, with the consequent high cumulative load, can delay or prevent ulcer healing. [145]

21. Prevention of diabetic ulcer formation

Lifetime prevalence of DFU development is estimated 25% [29,32]. Recurrence rate is also estimated to range from 28% at 12 months to 100% at 40 months. [146] At least 40% of amputations in diabetic patients can be prevented with a team approach to wound care.

Early detection of potential risk factors for ulceration can decrease the frequency of wound development. Diabetic patients should be educated regarding the importance of maintaining good glycemic control, wearing appropriate footwear, avoiding trauma, and performing frequent self-examination. They are also recommended to have their feet professionally examined at least annually (see table 9, according to the Foot Care Interest Group of the ADA) [55] to determine predisposing conditions to ulceration. In both self- and professionally-examining the foot, visual inspection of the bare foot should be performed in a well-lit room. The examination should include an assessment of the shoes; inappropriate footwear can be a contributing factor to the development of foot ulceration. In the visual inspection of the foot, the evaluator should check between the toes for the presence of ulceration or signs of infection. The presence of callus or nail abnormalities should be noted. Additionally, a temperature difference between feet is suggestive of vascular disease.

The foot should also be examined for deformities. The Charcot arthropathy is a commonly mentioned deformity in some affected diabetic patients.

Regardless ulcer treatment method, patients should slowly change to full activity and weight-bearing, using appropriate custom-made therapeutic footwear, while hyperglycemia, and neuron and vascular conditions are under a careful watch. Moreover, a proper patient and care-giver education, and regular foot care are of extreme importance in preventing DFU recurrence.

Author details

Bardia Farzamfar[1], Reza Nazari[2] and Saeed Bayanolhagh[3]

*Address all correspondence to: farzamfar@inoclon.com

1 Research and Development Department, G. Innovative Biotech Co., Alborz Province, Iran

2 Dept. Laboratory Medicine and Pathobiology, University of Toronto, Ontario, Canada

3 Saeed Bayanolhagh, Iranian Research Center for HIV/AIDS, Tehran University of Medical Sciences, Tehran, Iran

References

[1] Jeffcoate WJ, Harding KG. Diabetic foot ulcers. Lancet 2003 May 3;361(9368): 1545-1551.

[2] Boulton AJ. The diabetic foot: a global view. Diabetes Metab Res Rev 2000 Sep-Oct;16 Suppl 1:S2-5.

[3] Boulton AJ, Vileikyte L, Ragnarson-Tennvall G, Apelqvist J. The global burden of di-abetic foot disease. Lancet 2005 Nov 12;366(9498):1719-1724.

[4] Bartus CL, Margolis DJ. Reducing the incidence of foot ulceration and amputation in diabetes. Curr Diab Rep 2004 Dec;4(6):413-418.

[5] Margolis DJ, Malay DS, Hoffstad OJ, Leonard CE, MaCurdy T, Tan Y, et al. Economic Burden of Diabetic Foot Ulcers and Amputations: Data Points #3. Data Points Publi-cation Series Rockville (MD); 2011.

[6] Ragnarson Tennvall G, Apelqvist J. Health-economic consequences of diabetic foot lesions. Clin Infect Dis 2004 Aug 1;39 Suppl 2:S132-9.

[7] Lemaster JW, Reiber GE. Epidemiology and Economic Impact of Foot Ulcers. In: Boulton AJ, Cavanagh PR, Rayman G, editors. The Foot in Diabetes. 4th ed.: John Wi-ley & Sons; 2006. p. 3.

[8] Kernich CA. Patient and family fact sheet. Peripheral neuropathy. Neurologist 2001 Sep;7(5):315-316.

[9] Yagihashi S, Yamagishi S, Wada R. Pathology and pathogenetic mechanisms of dia-betic neuropathy: correlation with clinical signs and symptoms. Diabetes Res Clin Pract 2007 Sep;77 Suppl 1:S184-9.

[10] Peripheral Neuropathy. Available at: http://www.ncbi.nlm.nih.gov/pubmedhealth/ PMH0001619/.

[11] Zilliox L, Russell JW. Treatment of diabetic sensory polyneuropathy. Curr Treat Options Neurol 2011 Apr;13(2):143-159.

[12] Garces-Sanchez M, Laughlin RS, Dyck PJ, Engelstad JK, Norell JE, Dyck PJ. Painless diabetic motor neuropathy: a variant of diabetic lumbosacral radiculoplexus Neuropathy? Ann Neurol 2011 Jun;69(6):1043-1054.

[13] Real JT, Valls M, Ascaso P, Basanta ML, Viguer AA, Ascaso JF, et al. Risk factors associated to hospitalization in diabetic patients with foot ulcers. Med Clin (Barc) 2001 Nov 24;117(17):641-644.

[14] Armstrong DG, Lavery LA. Diabetic foot ulcers: prevention, diagnosis and classification. Am Fam Physician 1998 Mar 15;57(6):1325-32, 1337-8.

[15] Bowering CK. Diabetic foot ulcers. Pathophysiology, assessment, and therapy. Can Fam Physician 2001 May;47:1007-1016.

[16] Efrati S, Gall N, Bergan J, Fishlev G, Bass A, Berman S, et al. Hyperbaric oxygen, oxidative stress, NO bioavailability and ulcer oxygenation in diabetic patients. Undersea Hyperb Med 2009 Jan-Feb;36(1):1-12.

[17] Lavery LA, Peters EJ, Williams JR, Murdoch DP, Hudson A, Lavery DC, et al. Reevaluating the way we classify the diabetic foot: restructuring the diabetic foot risk classification system of the International Working Group on the Diabetic Foot. Diabetes Care 2008 Jan;31(1):154-156.

[18] Schaper NC, Nabuurs-Franssen MH. The diabetic foot: pathogenesis and clinical evaluation. Semin Vasc Med 2002 May;2(2):221-228.

[19] Frykberg RG. Diabetic foot ulcers: pathogenesis and management. Am Fam Physician 2002 Nov 1;66(9):1655-1662.

[20] Searles JM,Jr, Colen LB. Foot reconstruction in diabetes mellitus and peripheral vascular insufficiency. Clin Plast Surg 1991 Jul;18(3):467-483.

[21] Huijberts MS, Schaper NC, Schalkwijk CG. Advanced glycation end products and diabetic foot disease. Diabetes Metab Res Rev 2008 May-Jun;24 Suppl 1:S19-24.

[22] Zochodne DW. Diabetic polyneuropathy: an update. Curr Opin Neurol 2008 Oct; 21(5):527-533.

[23] Paraskevas KI, Baker DM, Pompella A, Mikhailidis DP. Does diabetes mellitus play a role in restenosis and patency rates following lower extremity peripheral arterial revascularization? A critical overview. Ann Vasc Surg 2008 May-Jun;22(3):481-491.

[24] Ziyadeh FN. The extracellular matrix in diabetic nephropathy. Am J Kidney Dis 1993 Nov;22(5):736-744.

[25] Jackle-Meyer I, Szukics B, Neubauer K, Metze V, Petzoldt R, Stolte H. Extracellular matrix proteins as early markers in diabetic nephropathy. Eur J Clin Chem Clin Biochem 1995 Apr;33(4):211-219.

[26] Mason RM, Wahab NA. Extracellular matrix metabolism in diabetic nephropathy. J Am Soc Nephrol 2003 May;14(5):1358-1373.

[27] Striker GE, Eastman RD, Striker LJ. Diabetic nephropathy: molecular analysis of extracellular matrix and clinical studies update. Nephrol Dial Transplant 1996;11 Suppl 5:58-61.

[28] Muller M, Trocme C, Lardy B, Morel F, Halimi S, Benhamou PY. Matrix metalloproteinases and diabetic foot ulcers: the ratio of MMP-1 to TIMP-1 is a predictor of wound healing. Diabet Med 2008 Apr;25(4):419-426.

[29] Nyamu PN, Otieno CF, Amayo EO, McLigeyo SO. Risk factors and prevalence of diabetic foot ulcers at Kenyatta National Hospital, Nairobi. East Afr Med J 2003 Jan; 80(1):36-43.

[30] Morrison WB, Ledermann HP. Work-up of the diabetic foot. Radiol Clin North Am 2002 Sep;40(5):1171-1192.

[31] Pecoraro RE, Reiber GE, Burgess EM. Pathways to diabetic limb amputation. Basis for prevention. Diabetes Care 1990 May;13(5):513-521.

[32] Singh N, Armstrong DG, Lipsky BA. Preventing foot ulcers in patients with diabetes. JAMA 2005 Jan 12;293(2):217-228.

[33] Tesfaye S, Selvarajah D. Advances in the epidemiology, pathogenesis and management of diabetic peripheral neuropathy. Diabetes Metab Res Rev 2012 Feb;28 Suppl 1:8-14.

[34] Boyko EJ, Ahroni JH, Stensel V, Forsberg RC, Davignon DR, Smith DG. A Prospective Study of Risk Factors for Diabetic Foot Ulcer. Diabetes Care 1999;22(7):1036-1042.

[35] Korzon-Burakowska A, Dziemidok P. Diabetic foot - the need for comprehensive multidisciplinary approach. Ann Agric Environ Med 2011 Dec;18(2):314-317.

[36] Crawford F, Inkster M, Kleijnen J, Fahey T. Predicting foot ulcers in patients with diabetes: a systematic review and meta-analysis. QJM 2007 Feb;100(2):65-86.

[37] Lavery LA, Armstrong DG, Wunderlich RP, Mohler MJ, Wendel CS, Lipsky BA. Risk factors for foot infections in individuals with diabetes. Diabetes Care 2006 Jun;29(6): 1288-1293.

[38] Al-Maskari F, El-Sadig M. Prevalence of risk factors for diabetic foot complications. BMC Fam Pract 2007 Oct 10;8:59.

[39] Tesfaye S, Chaturvedi N, Eaton SE, Ward JD, Manes C, Ionescu-Tirgoviste C, et al. Vascular risk factors and diabetic neuropathy. N Engl J Med 2005 Jan 27;352(4): 341-350.

[40] Clayton W, Elasy TM. A Review of the Pathophysiology, Classification, and Treatment of Foot Ulcers in Diabetic Patients. Clinical Diabetes 2009;27(2):52-58.

[41] Wagner FW,Jr. The diabetic foot. Orthopedics 1987 Jan;10(1):163-172.

[42] Oyibo SO, Jude EB, Tarawneh I, Nguyen HC, Harkless LB, Boulton AJ. A comparison of two diabetic foot ulcer classification systems: the Wagner and the University of Texas wound classification systems. Diabetes Care 2001 Jan;24(1):84-88.

[43] Treece KA, Macfarlane RM, Pound N, Game FL, Jeffcoate WJ. Validation of a system of foot ulcer classification in diabetes mellitus. Diabet Med 2004 Sep;21(9):987-991.

[44] Macfarlane RM, Jeffcoate WJ. Classification of Diabetic Foot Ulcers: The S(AD) SAD system. Diabetic Foot 1999;2:123-131.

[45] Cuzzell JZ. The new RYB color code. Am J Nurs 1988 Oct;88(10):1342-1346.

[46] Schaper NC. Diabetic foot ulcer classification system for research purposes: a progress report on criteria for including patients in research studies. Diabetes Metab Res Rev 2004 May-Jun;20 Suppl 1:S90-5.

[47] van Houtum WH, Rauwerda JA, Schaper NC, Bakker K. International Ulcer Classification for Research Purposes by The International Working Group on the Diabetic Foot. Proceedings of the 4th International Symposium on the Diabetic Foot. May 22–24, 2003 Noordwijkerhout, the Netherlands. Diab Metab Res Rev 2004;20(S1):S1.

[48] Younes NA, Albsoul AM. The DEPA scoring system and its correlation with the healing rate of diabetic foot ulcers. J Foot Ankle Surg 2004 Jul-Aug;43(4):209-213.

[49] Diegelmann RF, Evans MC. Wound healing: an overview of acute, fibrotic and delayed healing. Front Biosci 2004 Jan 1;9:283-289.

[50] Sheffield,P.J., Smith,A.P.S. Physiological and pharmacological basis of hyperbaric oxygen therapy. In: Bakker,D.J., Cramer,F.S., editor. Hyperbaric surgery: Flagstaff, AZ: Best Publishing Company; 2002. p. 63-109.

[51] Mantzaris NV, Webb S, Othmer HG. Mathematical modeling of tumor-induced angiogenesis. J Math Biol 2004 Aug;49(2):111-187.

[52] Bauer SM, Bauer RJ, Velazquez OC. Angiogenesis, vasculogenesis, and induction of healing in chronic wounds. Vasc Endovascular Surg 2005 Jul-Aug;39(4):293-306.

[53] Asahara T, Masuda H, Takahashi T, Kalka C, Pastore C, Silver M, et al. Bone marrow origin of endothelial progenitor cells responsible for postnatal vasculogenesis in physiological and pathological neovascularization. Circ Res 1999 Aug 6;85(3): 221-228.

[54] Byrne HM, Chaplain MA. Mathematical models for tumour angiogenesis: numerical simulations and nonlinear wave solutions. Bull Math Biol 1995 May;57(3):461-486.

[55] Boulton AJ, Armstrong DG, Albert SF, Frykberg RG, Hellman R, Kirkman MS, et al. Comprehensive foot examination and risk assessment: a report of the task force of the foot care interest group of the American Diabetes Association, with endorsement by the American Association of Clinical Endocrinologists. Diabetes Care 2008 Aug; 31(8):1679-1685.

[56] Khan NA, Rahim SA, Anand SS, Simel DL, Panju A. Does the clinical examination predict lower extremity peripheral arterial disease? JAMA 2006 Feb 1;295(5):536-546.

[57] American Diabetes Association. Peripheral arterial disease in people with diabetes. Diabetes Care 2003 Dec;26(12):3333-3341.

[58] International Working Group on the Diabetic Foot, International consensus on the diabetic foot and practical guidelines on the management and the prevention of the diabetic foot. Amsterdam, the Netherlands. 2011; Available at: (www.idf. org/ bookshop) or (www.diabeticfoot.nl).

[59] Apelqvist J, Armstrong DG, Lavery LA, Boulton AJ. Resource utilization and economic costs of care based on a randomized trial of vacuum-assisted closure therapy in the treatment of diabetic foot wounds. Am J Surg 2008 Jun;195(6):782-788.

[60] Murdoch DP, Armstrong DG, Dacus JB, Laughlin TJ, Morgan CB, Lavery LA. The natural history of great toe amputations. J Foot Ankle Surg 1997 May-Jun;36(3):204-8; discussion 256.

[61] Skoutas D, Papanas N, Georgiadis GS, Zervas V, Manes C, Maltezos E, et al. Risk factors for ipsilateral reamputation in patients with diabetic foot lesions. Int J Low Extrem Wounds 2009 Jun;8(2):69-74.

[62] Norgren L, Hiatt WR, Dormandy JA, Nehler MR, Harris KA, Fowkes FG, et al. Inter-society consensus for the management of peripheral arterial disease. Int Angiol 2007 Jun;26(2):81-157.

[63] Byrne RL, Nicholson ML, Woolford TJ, Callum KG. Factors influencing the healing of distal amputations performed for lower limb ischaemia. Br J Surg 1992 Jan;79(1): 73-75.

[64] Yeager RA, Moneta GL, Edwards JM, Williamson WK, McConnell DB, Taylor LM,Jr, et al. Predictors of outcome of forefoot surgery for ulceration and gangrene. Am J Surg 1998 May;175(5):388-390.

[65] Caruana MF, Bradbury AW, Adam DJ. The validity, reliability, reproducibility and extended utility of ankle to brachial pressure index in current vascular surgical practice. Eur J Vasc Endovasc Surg 2005 May;29(5):443-451.

[66] Faries PL, Teodorescu VJ, Morrissey NJ, Hollier LH, Marin ML. The role of surgical revascularization in the management of diabetic foot wounds. Am J Surg 2004 May; 187(5A):34S-37S.

[67] Lepantalo M, Biancari F, Tukiainen E. Never Amputate without Consultation of a Vascular Surgeon. Diabetes Metab Res Rev 2000;16(suppl 1):S27-S32.

[68] Teodorescu VJ, Chen C, Morrissey N, Faries PL, Marin ML, Hollier LH. Detailed protocol of ischemia and the use of noninvasive vascular laboratory testing in diabetic foot ulcers. Am J Surg 2004 May;187(5A):75S-80S.

[69] Jude EB, Unsworth PF. Optimal treatment of infected diabetic foot ulcers. Drugs Aging 2004;21(13):833-850.

[70] Shah DM, Darling RC,3rd, Chang BB, Fitzgerald KM, Paty PS, Leather RP. Long-term results of in situ saphenous vein bypass. Analysis of 2058 cases. Ann Surg 1995 Oct; 222(4):438-46; discussion 446-8.

[71] Edmonds M, Foster A. The use of antibiotics in the diabetic foot. Am J Surg 2004 May;187(5A):25S-28S.

[72] Lipsky BA, International consensus group on diagnosing and treating the infected diabetic foot. A report from the international consensus on diagnosing and treating the infected diabetic foot. Diabetes Metab Res Rev 2004 May-Jun;20 Suppl 1:S68-77.

[73] Jeffcoate WJ, Lipsky BA. Controversies in diagnosing and managing osteomyelitis of the foot in diabetes. Clin Infect Dis 2004 Aug 1;39 Suppl 2:S115-22.

[74] Game F. Management of osteomyelitis of the foot in diabetes mellitus. Nat Rev Endocrinol 2010 Jan;6(1):43-47.

[75] Sibbald RG, Orsted H, Schultz GS, Coutts P, Keast D, International Wound Bed Preparation Advisory Board, et al. Preparing the wound bed 2003: focus on infection and inflammation. Ostomy Wound Manage 2003 Nov;49(11):23-51.

[76] Badiavas EV, Abedi M, Butmarc J, Falanga V, Quesenberry P. Participation of bone marrow derived cells in cutaneous wound healing. J Cell Physiol 2003 Aug;196(2): 245-250.

[77] Saap LJ, Donohue K, Falanga V. Clinical classification of bioengineered skin use and its correlation with healing of diabetic and venous ulcers. Dermatol Surg 2004 Aug; 30(8):1095-1100.

[78] Brem H, Balledux J, Bloom T, Kerstein MD, Hollier L. Healing of diabetic foot ulcers and pressure ulcers with human skin equivalent: a new paradigm in wound healing. Arch Surg 2000 Jun;135(6):627-634.

[79] Smiell JM, Wieman TJ, Steed DL, Perry BH, Sampson AR, Schwab BH. Efficacy and safety of becaplermin (recombinant human platelet-derived growth factor-BB) in pa-

tients with nonhealing, lower extremity diabetic ulcers: a combined analysis of four randomized studies. Wound Repair Regen 1999 Sep-Oct;7(5):335-346.

[80] Steed DL. Clinical evaluation of recombinant human platelet-derived growth factor for the treatment of lower extremity ulcers. Plast Reconstr Surg 2006 Jun;117(7 Suppl):143S-149S; discussion 150S-151S.

[81] Venturi ML, Attinger CE, Mesbahi AN, Hess CL, Graw KS. Mechanisms and clinical applications of the vacuum-assisted closure (VAC) Device: a review. Am J Clin Dermatol 2005;6(3):185-194.

[82] Roeckl-Wiedmann I, Bennett M, Kranke P. Systematic review of hyperbaric oxygen in the management of chronic wounds. Br J Surg 2005 Jan;92(1):24-32.

[83] Thackham JA, McElwain DL, Long RJ. The use of hyperbaric oxygen therapy to treat chronic wounds: A review. Wound Repair Regen 2008 May-Jun;16(3):321-330.

[84] Steed DL, Donohoe D, Webster MW, Lindsley L. Effect of extensive debridement and treatment on the healing of diabetic foot ulcers. Diabetic Ulcer Study Group. J Am Coll Surg 1996 Jul;183(1):61-64.

[85] Wolff H, Hansson C. Larval therapy--an effective method of ulcer debridement. Clin Exp Dermatol 2003 Mar;28(2):134-137.

[86] Horobin AJ, Shakesheff KM, Pritchard DI. Maggots and wound healing: an investigation of the effects of secretions from Lucilia sericata larvae upon the migration of human dermal fibroblasts over a fibronectin-coated surface. Wound Repair Regen 2005 Jul-Aug;13(4):422-433.

[87] Rosales A, Vazquez JR, Short B, Kimbriel HR, Claxton MJ, Nixon BP, et al. Use of a maggot motility index to evaluate survival of therapeutic larvae. J Am Podiatr Med Assoc 2004 Jul-Aug;94(4):353-355.

[88] Armstrong DG, Salas P, Short B, Martin BR, Kimbriel HR, Nixon BP, et al. Maggot therapy in "lower-extremity hospice" wound care: fewer amputations and more antibiotic-free days. J Am Podiatr Med Assoc 2005 May-Jun;95(3):254-257.

[89] Farzamfar B, Madani H, Gharibdoust F, Farhadi M, Novitsky YA, Khorramkhorshid HR, et al, inventors. Anonymous Herbal Extract for Treatment of Chronic Wounds. USA patent US 2010/0233305 A1. 2010 Apr 23, 2010.

[90] Bahrami A, Kamali K, Ali-Asgharzadeh A, Hosseini P, Heshmat R, Khorram Khorshid HR, et al. Clinical application of oral form of ANGIPARS™ and in combination with topical form as a new treatment for diabetic foot ulcers: A randomized clinical trial. Daru 2008;16(Suppl. 1):41-48.

[91] Larijani B, Heshmat R, Bahrami A, Delshad H, Ranjbar Omrani G, Mohammad K, et al. Effects of intravenous Semelil (ANGIPARS) on diabetic foot ulcers healing: A multicenter clinical trial. Daru 2008;16(Suppl. 1):35-40.

[92] Ebrahimi M, Bakhshayeshi S, Heshmat R, Shahbazi SA,M., Peimani M, Khushechin
      G, et al. Post marketing surveillance on safety and effectiveness of ANGIPARS in
      treatment of diabetic foot ulcers. Daru 2009;17(Suppl. 1):45-49.

[93] Larijani B, Hasani Ranjbar S. Overview of diabetic foot; novel treatments in diabetic
      foot ulcer. Daru 2008;16(Suppl. 1):1-6.

[94] Shamimi Nouri K, Heshmat R, Karimian R, Nasli E, Larijani B, Novitsky YA, et al.
      Intravenous Semelil (ANGIPARS™) as a novel therapy for pressure Ulcers: A
      randomized clinical trial. Daru 2008;16(Suppl. 1):49-53.

[95] Shamimi Nouri K, Karimian R, Nasli E, Kamali K, Chaman R, Farhadi M, et al. Topi-
      cal application of Semelil (ANGIPARS™) in treatment of pressure ulcers: A random-
      ized clinical trial. Daru 2008;16(Suppl. 1):54-57.

[96] Mousavi-Jazi M, Aslroosta H, Moayer AR, Baeeri M, Abdollahi M. Effects of Angi-
      pars on oxidative inflammatory indices in a murine model of periodontitis. Daru
      2010;18(4):260-264.

[97] Murphy PS, Evans GR. Advances in wound healing: a review of current wound heal-
      ing products. Plast Surg Int 2012;2012:190436.

[98] Argenta LC, Morykwas MJ. Vacuum-assisted closure: a new method for wound con-
      trol and treatment: clinical experience. Ann Plast Surg 1997 Jun;38(6):563-76; discus-
      sion 577.

[99] Buttenschoen K, Fleischmann W, Haupt U, Kinzl L, Buttenschoen DC. The influence
      of vacuum-assisted closure on inflammatory tissue reactions in the postoperative
      course of ankle fractures. Foot Ankle Surg 2001;7(3):165-173.

[100] Moues CM, van den Bemd GJ, Meerding WJ, Hovius SE. An economic evaluation of
      the use of TNP on full-thickness wounds. J Wound Care 2005 May;14(5):224-227.

[101] Leininger BE, Rasmussen TE, Smith DL, Jenkins DH, Coppola C. Experience with
      wound VAC and delayed primary closure of contaminated soft tissue injuries in
      Iraq. J Trauma 2006 Nov;61(5):1207-1211.

[102] Braakenburg A, Obdeijn MC, Feitz R, van Rooij IA, van Griethuysen AJ, Klinkenbijl
      JH. The clinical efficacy and cost effectiveness of the vacuum-assisted closure techni-
      que in the management of acute and chronic wounds: a randomized controlled trial.
      Plast Reconstr Surg 2006 Aug;118(2):390-7; discussion 398-400.

[103] Park CA, Defranzo AJ, Marks MW, Molnar JA. Outpatient reconstruction using inte-
      gra* and subatmospheric pressure. Ann Plast Surg 2009 Feb;62(2):164-169.

[104] Hurd T, Chadwick P, Cote J, Cockwill J, Mole TR, Smith JM. Impact of gauze-based
      NPWT on the patient and nursing experience in the treatment of challenging
      wounds. Int Wound J 2010 Dec;7(6):448-455.

[105] Ubbink DT, Westerbos SJ, Evans D, Land L, Vermeulen H. Topical negative pressure for treating chronic wounds. Cochrane Database Syst Rev 2008 Jul 16;(3) (3):CD001898.

[106] Peinemann F, Sauerland S. Negative-pressure wound therapy: systematic review of randomized controlled trials. Dtsch Arztebl Int 2011 Jun;108(22):381-389.

[107] Armstrong DG, Lavery LA, Diabetic Foot Study Consortium. Negative pressure wound therapy after partial diabetic foot amputation: a multicentre, randomised controlled trial. Lancet 2005 Nov 12;366(9498):1704-1710.

[108] Program and abstracts. Undersea and Hyperbaric Medical Society annual scientific meeting. 23-27 June 1992, Bethesda, Maryland. Undersea Biomed Res 1992;19 Suppl: 1-161.

[109] Eskes AM, Ubbink DT, Lubbers MJ, Lucas C, Vermeulen H. Hyperbaric oxygen therapy: solution for difficult to heal acute wounds? Systematic review. World J Surg 2011 Mar;35(3):535-542.

[110] Faglia E, Favales F, Aldeghi A, Calia P, Quarantiello A, Oriani G, et al. Adjunctive systemic hyperbaric oxygen therapy in treatment of severe prevalently ischemic diabetic foot ulcer. A randomized study. Diabetes Care 1996 Dec;19(12):1338-1343.

[111] Barnes RC. Point: hyperbaric oxygen is beneficial for diabetic foot wounds. Clin Infect Dis 2006 Jul 15;43(2):188-192.

[112] Goldman RJ. Hyperbaric oxygen therapy for wound healing and limb salvage: a systematic review. PM R 2009 May;1(5):471-489.

[113] Hilton JR, Williams DT, Beuker B, Miller DR, Harding KG. Wound dressings in diabetic foot disease. Clin Infect Dis 2004 Aug 1;39 Suppl 2:S100-3.

[114] Foster AV, Eaton C, McConville DO, Edmonds ME. Application of OpSite film: a new and effective treatment of painful diabetic neuropathy. Diabet Med 1994 Oct; 11(8):768-772.

[115] Morin RJ, Tomaselli NL. Interactive dressings and topical agents. Clin Plast Surg 2007 Oct;34(4):643-658.

[116] Khundkar R, Malic C, Burge T. Use of Acticoat dressings in burns: what is the evidence? Burns 2010 Sep;36(6):751-758.

[117] Atiyeh BS, Costagliola M, Hayek SN, Dibo SA. Effect of silver on burn wound infection control and healing: review of the literature. Burns 2007 Mar;33(2):139-148.

[118] Stanford W, Rappole BW, Fox CL,Jr. Clinical experience with silver sulfadiazine, a new topical agent for control of pseudomonas infections in burns. J Trauma 1969 May;9(5):377-388.

[119] Cruciani M, Lipsky BA, Mengoli C, de Lalla F. Are granulocyte colony-stimulating factors beneficial in treating diabetic foot infections?: A meta-analysis. Diabetes Care 2005 Feb;28(2):454-460.

[120] Cianfarani F, Tommasi R, Failla CM, Viviano MT, Annessi G, Papi M, et al. Granulo-cyte/macrophage colony-stimulating factor treatment of human chronic ulcers promotes angiogenesis associated with de novo vascular endothelial growth factor transcription in the ulcer bed. Br J Dermatol 2006 Jan;154(1):34-41.

[121] Sato N, Kashima K, Tanaka Y, Shimizu H, Mori M. Effect of granulocyte-colony stimulating factor on generation of oxygen-derived free radicals and myeloperoxidase activity in neutrophils from poorly controlled NIDDM patients. Diabetes 1997 Jan; 46(1):133-137.

[122] Margolis DJ, Bartus C, Hoffstad O, Malay S, Berlin JA. Effectiveness of recombinant human platelet-derived growth factor for the treatment of diabetic neuropathic foot ulcers. Wound Repair Regen 2005 Nov-Dec;13(6):531-536.

[123] Steed DL. Clinical evaluation of recombinant human platelet-derived growth factor for the treatment of lower extremity diabetic ulcers. Diabetic Ulcer Study Group. J Vasc Surg 1995 Jan;21(1):71-8; discussion 79-81.

[124] Blumberg SN, Berger A, Hwang I., Pastar I, Warren SM, Chen W. The role of stem cells in the treatment of diabetic foot ulcers. Diabetes Res Clin Pract 2012 Apr;96(1): 1-9.

[125] Tran TC, Kimura K, Nagano M, Yamashita T, Ohneda K, Sugimori H, et al. Identification of human placenta-derived mesenchymal stem cells involved in re-endothelialization. J Cell Physiol 2011 Jan;226(1):224-235.

[126] Lu D, Chen B, Liang Z, Deng W, Jiang Y, Li S, et al. Comparison of bone marrow mesenchymal stem cells with bone marrow-derived mononuclear cells for treatment of diabetic critical limb ischemia and foot ulcer: a double-blind, randomized, controlled trial. Diabetes Res Clin Pract 2011 Apr;92(1):26-36.

[127] Lee MJ, Kim J, Lee KI, Shin JM, Chae JI, Chung HM. Enhancement of wound healing by secretory factors of endothelial precursor cells derived from human embryonic stem cells. Cytotherapy 2011 Feb;13(2):165-178.

[128] Falanga V, Iwamoto S, Chartier M, Yufit T, Butmarc J, Kouttab N, et al. Autologous bone marrow-derived cultured mesenchymal stem cells delivered in a fibrin spray accelerate healing in murine and human cutaneous wounds. Tissue Eng 2007 Jun; 13(6):1299-1312.

[129] Prochazka V, Gumulec J, Chmelova J, Klement P, Klement GL, Jonszta T, et al. Autologous bone marrow stem cell transplantation in patients with end-stage chronical critical limb ischemia and diabetic foot. Vnitr Lek 2009 Mar;55(3):173-178.

[130] Capla JM, Grogan RH, Callaghan MJ, Galiano RD, Tepper OM, Ceradini DJ, et al. Diabetes impairs endothelial progenitor cell-mediated blood vessel formation in response to hypoxia. Plast Reconstr Surg 2007 Jan;119(1):59-70.

[131] Ehrenreich M, Ruszczak Z. Update on tissue-engineered biological dressings. Tissue Eng 2006 Sep;12(9):2407-2424.

[132] Alexiadou K, Doupis J. Management of diabetic foot ulcers. Diabetes Ther 2012 Nov; 3(1):4.

[133] Edmonds M, European and Australian Apligraf Diabetic Foot Ulcer Study Group. Apligraf in the treatment of neuropathic diabetic foot ulcers. Int J Low Extrem Wounds 2009 Mar;8(1):11-18.

[134] Moustafa M, Bullock AJ, Creagh FM, Heller S, Jeffcoate W, Game F, et al. Randomized, controlled, single-blind study on use of autologous keratinocytes on a transfer dressing to treat nonhealing diabetic ulcers. Regen Med 2007 Nov;2(6):887-902.

[135] Mahmoud SM, Mohamed AA, Mahdi SE, Ahmed ME. Split-skin graft in the management of diabetic foot ulcers. J Wound Care 2008 Jul;17(7):303-306.

[136] Uccioli L, Giurato L, Ruotolo V, Ciavarella A, Grimaldi MS, Piaggesi A, et al. Two-step autologous grafting using HYAFF scaffolds in treating difficult diabetic foot ulcers: results of a multicenter, randomized controlled clinical trial with long-term follow-up. Int J Low Extrem Wounds 2011 Jun;10(2):80-85.

[137] Moustafa M, Simpson C, Glover M, Dawson RA, Tesfaye S, Creagh FM, et al. A new autologous keratinocyte dressing treatment for non-healing diabetic neuropathic foot ulcers. Diabet Med 2004 Jul;21(7):786-789.

[138] Niezgoda JA, Van Gils CC, Frykberg RG, Hodde JP. Randomized clinical trial comparing OASIS Wound Matrix to Regranex Gel for diabetic ulcers. Adv Skin Wound Care 2005 Jun;18(5 Pt 1):258-266.

[139] Martin BR, Sangalang M, Wu S, Armstrong DG. Outcomes of allogenic acellular matrix therapy in treatment of diabetic foot wounds: an initial experience. Int Wound J 2005 Jun;2(2):161-165.

[140] Masoompour SM, Bagheri MH, Borhani Haghighi A, Novitsky YA, Sadeghi B, Gharibdoust F, et al. Effect of ANGIPARS™, a new herbal drug on diabetic foot ulcer: A phase 2 clinical study. DARU 2008;16(Suppl. 1):31-34.

[141] Rose Pharmed Biotechnology Co. Available at: www.rosepharmed.com.

[142] Petre M, Tokar P, Kostar D, Cavanagh PR. Revisiting the total contact cast: maximizing off-loading by wound isolation. Diabetes Care 2005 Apr;28(4):929-930.

[143] Armstrong DG, Lavery LA, Kimbriel HR, Nixon BP, Boulton AJ. Activity patterns of patients with diabetic foot ulceration: patients with active ulceration may not adhere to a standard pressure off-loading regimen. Diabetes Care 2003 Sep;26(9):2595-2597.

[144] Caravaggi C, Faglia E, De Giglio R, Mantero M, Quarantiello A, Sommariva E, et al. Effectiveness and safety of a nonremovable fiberglass off-bearing cast versus a therapeutic shoe in the treatment of neuropathic foot ulcers: a randomized study. Diabetes Care 2000 Dec;23(12):1746-1751.

[145] Maluf KS, Mueller MJ. Novel Award 2002. Comparison of physical activity and cumulative plantar tissue stress among subjects with and without diabetes mellitus and a history of recurrent plantar ulcers. Clin Biomech (Bristol, Avon) 2003 Aug;18(7): 567-575.

[146] Mantey I, Foster AV, Spencer S, Edmonds ME. Why do foot ulcers recur in diabetic patients? Diabet Med 1999 Mar;16(3):245-249.

Permissions

The contributors of this book come from diverse backgrounds, making this book a truly international effort. This book will bring forth new frontiers with its revolutionizing research information and detailed analysis of the nascent developments around the world.

We would like to thank Dr. Alexander A. Vitin, MD, Ph.D, for lending his expertise to make the book truly unique. He has played a crucial role in the development of this book. Without his invaluable contribution this book wouldn't have been possible. He has made vital efforts to compile up to date information on the varied aspects of this subject to make this book a valuable addition to the collection of many professionals and students.

This book was conceptualized with the vision of imparting up-to-date information and advanced data in this field. To ensure the same, a matchless editorial board was set up. Every individual on the board went through rigorous rounds of assessment to prove their worth. After which they invested a large part of their time researching and compiling the most relevant data for our readers. Conferences and sessions were held from time to time between the editorial board and the contributing authors to present the data in the most comprehensible form. The editorial team has worked tirelessly to provide valuable and valid information to help people across the globe.

Every chapter published in this book has been scrutinized by our experts. Their significance has been extensively debated. The topics covered herein carry significant findings which will fuel the growth of the discipline. They may even be implemented as practical applications or may be referred to as a beginning point for another development. Chapters in this book were first published by InTech; hereby published with permission under the Creative Commons Attribution License or equivalent.

The editorial board has been involved in producing this book since its inception. They have spent rigorous hours researching and exploring the diverse topics which have resulted in the successful publishing of this book. They have passed on their knowledge of decades through this book. To expedite this challenging task, the publisher supported the team at every step. A small team of assistant editors was also appointed to further simplify the editing procedure and attain best results for the readers.

Our editorial team has been hand-picked from every corner of the world. Their multi-ethnicity adds dynamic inputs to the discussions which result in innovative outcomes. These outcomes are then further discussed with the researchers and contributors who give their valuable feedback and opinion regarding the same. The feedback is then collaborated with the researches and they are edited in a comprehensive manner to aid the understanding of the subject.

Apart from the editorial board, the designing team has also invested a significant amount of their time in understanding the subject and creating the most relevant covers. They scrutinized every image to scout for the most suitable representation of the subject and create an appropriate cover for the book.

The publishing team has been involved in this book since its early stages. They were actively engaged in every process, be it collecting the data, connecting with the contributors or procuring relevant information. The team has been an ardent support to the editorial, designing and production team. Their endless efforts to recruit the best for this project, has resulted in the accomplishment of this book. They are a veteran in the field of academics and their pool of knowledge is as vast as their experience in printing. Their expertise and guidance has proved useful at every step. Their uncompromising quality standards have made this book an exceptional effort. Their encouragement from time to time has been an inspiration for everyone.

The publisher and the editorial board hope that this book will prove to be a valuable piece of knowledge for researchers, students, practitioners and scholars across the globe.

List of Contributors

P.E. Ekanem and Ekanem P.
Department of Anatomy, Kampala International University, Western Campus, Ishaka, Bushenyi, Uganda

O.E. Dafiewhare
Department of Internal Medicine, Kampala International University, Western Campus, Ishaka, Bushenyi, Uganda

A.M. Ajayi
Department of Pharmacology, Kampala International University, Western Campus, Ishaka, Bushenyi, Uganda

R. Ekanem
Department of Nursing Science, Kampala International University, Western Campus, Ishaka, Bushenyi, Uganda

W. Agwu and Agwu E
Department of Microbiology, Kampala International University, Western Campus, Ishaka, Bushenyi, Uganda

Ezeonwumelu J.O.C.
Department of Clinical and Bio-pharmacy, Kampala International University, Western Campus, Ishaka, Bushenyi, Uganda

Okoruwa G.
School of Pharmacy, Kampala International University, Western Campus, Ishaka, Bushenyi, Uganda

Shaban A.
Department of Surgery, Kampala International University, Western Campus, Ishaka, Bushenyi, Uganda

F. Santosa
Klinik Angiologi & Kardiologi "Waringin Medika", Jakarta, Indonesia

K. Kröger
Department of Angiology, HELIOS Klinikum Krefeld, Germany

Slim Jarboui and Abdelwaheb Hlel
Faculté de Medecine de Sousse, Department of General Surgery- Hospital of SidiBouzid, University of Medicine of Sousse, Tunisia

Alifa Daghfous and Lamia Rezgui Marhoul
Faculté de Medecine de Sousse, Department of Radiology- Trauma Center of Ben Arous, University of Medicine of Sousse, Tunisia

Bardia Farzamfar
Research and Development Department, G. Innovative Biotech Co., Alborz Province, Iran

Reza Nazari
Dept. Laboratory Medicine and Pathobiology, University of Toronto, Ontario, Canada

Saeed Bayanolhagh
Iranian Research Center for HIV/AIDS, Tehran University of Medical Sciences, Tehran, Iran